T0144851

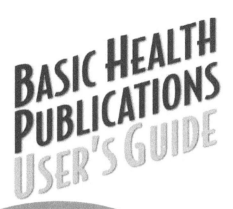

BASIC HEALTH PUBLICATIONS USER'S GUIDE

TO ECHINACEA AND OTHER COLD & FLU FIGHTERS

How Vitamins and Herbs Can Get You Back on Your Feet Safely and Quickly.

LAUREL VUKOVIC, M.S.W.

JACK CHALLEM Series Editor

The information contained in this book is based upon the research and personal and professional experiences of the author. It is not intended as a substitute for consulting with your physician or other healthcare provider. Any attempt to diagnose and treat an illness should be done under the direction of a healthcare professional.

The publisher does not advocate the use of any particular healthcare protocol but believes the information in this book should be available to the public. The publisher and author are not responsible for any adverse effects or consequences resulting from the use of the suggestions, preparations, or procedures discussed in this book. Should the reader have any questions concerning the appropriateness of any procedures or preparations mentioned, the author and the publisher strongly suggest consulting a professional healthcare advisor.

Series Editor: Jack Challem
Editor: Gina Friedlander
Typesetter: Gary A. Rosenberg
Series Cover Designer: Mike Stromberg

Basic Health Publications User's Guides are published by Basic Health Publications, Inc.

ISBN: 978-1-59120-084-0 (Pbk.)
ISBN: 978-1-68162-851-6 (Hardcover)

CONTENTS

Introduction, 1

1. How Colds and Flus "Catch You", 3

2. Simple Ways to Strengthen Your Immune System, 14

3. Immune-Boosting Herbs: Echinacea and Astragalus, 21

4. Virus-Fighting Herbs: Elderberry and Garlic, 36

5. Virus-Fighting Nutrients: Vitamin C, N-acetylcysteine, and Zinc, 46

6. Why You Shouldn't Take Drugs for Colds and Flus, 55

7. Home Remedies for Colds and Flus, 60

8. How to Buy and Use Supplements and Herbs, 73

Conclusion, 79

Selected References, 81

Other Books and Resources, 83

Index, 85

INTRODUCTION

Chances are, you're going to come down with a cold or flu this year. If you're like most people, you have an assortment of pain relievers, decongestants, cough syrups, and other over-the-counter and prescription drugs that you've collected for easing the misery of a cold or flu.

But did you know that although such medicines may give you temporary relief from cold and flu symptoms, studies have shown that taking such drugs actually prolongs the length of time that you will be sick? Instead of getting well faster, you could be sick for *twice* as long as if you took nothing at all. In addition, many of the medications for colds and flus have unpleasant and even hazardous side effects, ranging from drowsiness to heart rhythm disturbances.

There is another serious drawback to using drugs. The antibiotic prescriptions that are frequently handed out for treating colds and flus are now recognized as a primary factor in the evolution of killer germs—bacteria that are drug-resistant and highly dangerous.

Fortunately, there are safe and effective alternatives to pharmaceutical drugs. Herbs such as echinacea, elderberry, astragalus, and garlic are key players in helping to strengthen the body's natural defenses against the viruses that cause colds and flus. And nutrients such as vitamin C, N-acetylcysteine, and zinc provide essential support to your body's immune system. Using herbs and nutritional supplements is radically different from using medications that simply mask the symptoms of a cold or flu. When you use natural remedies, you are enhancing your immune function, building your resistance to invading micro-organisms, and improving your overall health.

In this book, you'll learn how cold and flu viruses operate, and how you can avoid them. You'll also discover how you can enhance your body's innate ability to fend off viruses. And if you do occasionally come down with a cold or flu, you'll learn how to relieve the uncomfortable symptoms naturally, safely, and effectively and speed your recovery.

CHAPTER 1

How Colds and Flus "Catch You"

Colds and flus are the most common illnesses that plague humankind. Statistically, you're likely to come down with a cold up to four times this year (young children can catch up to a dozen colds per year), and according to the United States Centers for Disease Control and Prevention (CDC), between 35 and 50 million Americans are striken with the flu each year. Antibiotics are useless against these illnesses because they are caused by viruses, not by bacteria. Over-the-counter medications offer little more than temporary relief from symptoms and may actually do more harm than good.

But there are many things that you can do to prevent colds and flus. Understanding how the viruses operate is a good starting point for gaining the knowledge that will give you the upper hand over these annoying and debilitating illnesses.

The Difference Between Colds and Flus

Colds and flus have a lot in common, but there are also some significant differences. Figuring out which is which can help you to identify the remedies that best suit your needs.

Colds are upper respiratory illnesses that can be caused by more than 200 different viruses. Although each virus actually causes a different cold, because the symptoms are so similar we think of them as a single illness—the common cold. The symptoms of a cold typically begin with minor throat irritation and progress, often within a matter of hours, to a full-blown sore throat, runny nose, nasal congestion, sneezing, and coughing. The nasal discharge that accompanies a cold is usually clear and runny for the first couple of days and then becomes thick and turns greenish yellow. The residual cough and congestion of a cold can last for one to two weeks and sometimes even longer. A fever accompanies only about 10 percent of colds and tends to be very mild in adults. In children, fever associated with a cold may run as high as 103°F for a couple of days.

Although colds rarely cause serious complications, they can lay the groundwork for subsequent problems such as sinus or middle-ear infections. Colds can also exacerbate asthma and can sometimes be followed by lingering bronchial irritation or infections. Young children are especially susceptible to painful middle-ear infections, which are linked to the cold virus. Sinusitis more commonly affects adults and is an infection of the sinus cavities with symptoms of nasal congestion, pressure or pain in the sinuses, headache, and a yellowish-green mucous discharge.

More serious respiratory infections such as bronchitis and pneumonia can also follow a cold, especially for the elderly or those with lowered immunity. Bronchitis is an infection of the bronchi, the tubes that carry air to the lungs. Symptoms include a persistent phlegm-producing cough and breathlessness. Acute bronchitis is usually caused by a virus and can last from a few days to two weeks or longer.

Bronchitis
An infection of the tubes that carry air to the lungs.

Pneumonia is a potentially dangerous viral or

bacterial infection of one or both lungs. The symptoms include fever, chills, breathlessness, chest pain, and a cough that produces yellow or green phlegm, sometimes tinged with blood.

Pneumonia
A bacterial or viral infection of the lungs.

In contrast to a cold, the flu (medically termed influenza) is a respiratory illness that is caused by a specific virus and is always more severe than a cold. The symptoms of flu include a high fever (up to 104°F), sore throat, coughing, headache, fatigue, nasal congestion, and aching joints and muscles. The intense symptoms of the flu generally last for about a week with residual fatigue lingering for an additional week or two.

Influenza (flu)
Respiratory illness caused by a virus.

The most serious complication of the flu is pneumonia, which can develop about five days following a bout with influenza in susceptible people. Although pneumonia is unlikely in healthy adults, the risk is very high for certain groups of people, including the elderly, very young children, and those with weakened immune systems. In addition, people with heart or lung diseases are at a higher risk of dying from the flu.

Why the Flu Can Be Deadly

Although for most of us influenza means just an uncomfortable few days in bed, there's no doubt that it can be deadly. As recently as 1918, a flu epidemic killed more than 25 million people around the world. The CDC estimates that in a typical year more than 100,000 people in the United States are hospitalized as a result of the flu, and close to 20,000 people die from the virus and its complications, such as pneumonia. However, if the strain of influenza is especially virulent, the number of hospitalizations and deaths skyrockets. Influenza epidemics are most dangerous when they involve a flu virus to which most people have not been previously exposed—such as a new strain of the flu or one that has not been circulating for many decades. In such cases, the virus can quickly spread throughout the world and is referred to as a pandemic.

Pandemic
A worldwide epidemic.

Knowing a little about how flu viruses operate can help you understand how to best protect yourself against these troublemaking microorgan-isms. In simple scientific terms, flu viruses are chains of genetic material encased in protein membranes, surrounded by a fatty envelope embedded with glycoprotein spikes. There are three recognized strains of influenza, determined by whether they have one or two protein membranes and the makeup of the glycoprotein spikes.

The three types of influenza viruses are identified as A, B, and C. The most common types are A and B. The type A virus is the one that is the most prevalent, is constantly mutating, and is the type that has caused the most devastating worldwide epidemics. The type A virus also is generally concentrated in large population centers and can infect animals as well as humans. The type B virus causes a milder flu and only infects humans, but it can also cause epidemics. Type C viruses cause mild illness and have never created an epidemic.

Our immune systems are generally able to protect us from invading microorganisms by recognizing the invader—in this case, a flu virus—and creating an antibody to the virus. But flu virus-es are able to quickly change their appearance and thus evade the surveillance of the immune system. Although flu viruses have been

Antibody
A protein made by the immune sys-tem that disables viruses.

around forever, our immune systems haven't been able to build up immunity to them because the viruses are constantly mutating. Consequently, each new strain of the flu causes the immune system to launch a full-scale attack against the virus, but that only provides immunity to that particular virus. Once inside the body, the virus multiplies by entering healthy cells and taking over, using the cell to make new virus particles. Another reason that flu viruses are so problematic is that they are highly contagious and generally have an incubation period of 24 to 72 hours. This means that it takes one to three days for symptoms to appear, giving the virus ample opportunity to spread.

What about Flu Vaccines?

Conventional healthcare professionals generally recommend the flu vaccine as the best way of preventing influenza. But many natural health practitioners aren't as quick to recommend flu shots for everyone. While there are some people who should be vaccinated, including the elderly and those with heart or lung disease or lowered immunity, most natural health practitioners don't advise the flu shot for healthy adults. Some practitioners are concerned that overimmunization can lead to problems with allergies and autoimmune disorders and advise to avoid flu shots unless you fall into a high-risk category. The CDC has recently recommended that children between the ages of six months and two years be immunized because they are also at risk of severe complications from the flu. However, because the safety of the flu vaccine has not been proven for this age group, if you have young children, discuss the issue with your pediatrician.

To confuse the issue further, getting immunized against the virus doesn't guarantee that you won't still come down with the flu. That's because the experts in the United States Food and Drug Administration (FDA) who select the combination of viruses early each year for the flu vaccine are simply making their best guess as to which viruses are most likely to cause epidemics later that year. Although vaccines are monitored carefully by the FDA, the Centers for Disease Control, and the World Health Organization, the choice of which viruses to include is always a roll of the dice. The virus strains used in making the vaccine are selected months before the flu season hits, and it's not uncommon for one or more of the strains circulating at the time the vaccine is formulated to mutate prior to flu season.

Flu vaccines are made from inactivated flu viruses. When the dead viruses are injected into your body, they stimulate an immune reaction to those particular strains of the flu. Because the virus is cultured in eggs to produce the vaccine, you should consult with your physician before getting the flu shot if you are allergic to eggs.

The flu season typically begins in November and lasts until March, so if you decide to get a flu shot, you should do so between October and mid-November to give your immune system time to build immunity to the flu. You should also be sure to get a good night's sleep before you go for a flu vaccine, according to a study in the September 2002 issue of the *Journal of the American Medical Association* that showed that the protective effects are decreased by sleep deprivation. The most common side effects of a flu vaccine are soreness from the injection and a slight fever that can last for a couple of days.

Whether or not you choose to get a flu shot, you can greatly increase your odds of escaping the flu by taking steps to strengthen your natural

immunity and by following commonsense precautions to avoid exposure to the flu virus.

How Viruses Infect You

Viruses are spread either through the air or by
direct contact. You can become infected by inhal-
ing virus particles that are expelled when an
infected person coughs or sneezes. You can also
pick up a virus by touching the hand of a person
who is sick or by touching a surface (such as a
doorknob, countertop, keyboard, or telephone)
that an infected person has recently touched. If
you then touch your nose or eyes (which most of
us do far more often than we realize), you give
the virus access to your body.

The virus then penetrates the protective
mucus in the nasal passages and sets up housekeeping in the throat. Once you start to notice
symptoms, the virus has already been replicating
for about ten to twelve hours. The resulting
inflammation from the virus brings a rush of
blood with infection-fighting white blood cells to
the area and causes the sore throat that is characteristic of a cold or flu. The body mounts a
fever to kill the virus, extra mucus is produced to
flush out the virus, and coughing and sneezing
help to expel the virus. As unpleasant as the
symptoms of a cold or flu can be, you should
keep in mind that they are caused by the body's
attack on the virus. Suppressing these symptoms
with drugs interferes with your body's efforts to
heal and is actually counterproductive. Further-
more, drugs don't fight the virus, nor do they
strengthen your immunity.

General Tips for Preventing Colds and Flus

A few simple precautions can greatly improve
your odds of fending off cold and flu viruses.

Most important is to wash your hands frequently, especially after spending time in public places or after shaking hands with someone. As much as possible, avoid close contact with anyone suffering from a cold or flu.

The greatest concentration of cold viruses live in the nose. When a person who has a cold touches his or her nose and then shakes your hand, the virus is easily transferred to your nasal passages if you touch your nose or your eyes (the tear ducts in the eyes are connected by a tube to the nasal passages). Doorknobs and telephones are also repositories for cold viruses lying in wait for unwitting victims. The simplest solution is to wash your hands frequently with soap and water and to consciously avoid touching your nose and eyes.

Although most colds and flus occur during the winter, it doesn't really have much to do with the cold weather. However, dry winter air—including the dryness created by indoor heating—parches the mucous membranes of the nose and throat, which makes them more susceptible to viruses. In addition, people tend to spend more time in-doors during the winter and are exposed to more people and higher concentrations of viruses.

Keeping the air in your home and office from becoming too dry will help to thwart cold and flu viruses. You can add moisture to the air by using a humidifier or with simple measures, such as placing a bowl of water on top of a radiator, simmering a pot of water uncovered on the stove for an hour or two, or leaving the bathroom door open during a shower to allow the steam to escape into the house.

If someone in your household is sick, have him or her sleep in a separate room, provide disposable tissues instead of cloth handkerchiefs, and make sure the used tissues are disposed of right away. Use a natural disinfectant spray that contains antimicrobial essential oils such as eucalyptus and lavender to keep phones, countertops, and other solid surfaces clean.

Natural Antimicrobial Protection

Antimicrobial chemicals are currently being used with abandon and are included in everything from skin cleansers to kitchen sponges. While protecting ourselves from disease-causing microorganisms is a good idea, it's a dangerous trend to attempt wholesale eradication of germs. One serious problem is that harmful microbes can become chemically resistant and mutate into stronger versions of themselves. In addition, instead of focusing on trying to create a sterile environment, which is impossible anyway in the average home, it makes more sense to concentrate on strengthening our immune systems by eating well, getting enough exercise and rest, and taking immune-building supplements and herbs.

Antimicrobe
A substance that kills disease-causing organisms.

However, there's no question that cleanliness is essential for preventing infection by disease-causing microorganisms. The usual precautions that you have heard many times make good common sense—wash your hands often, especially after being in public places and before preparing or eating food. But instead of using a chemical, antimicrobial soap, you can buy or make a liquid antiseptic hand soap with essential oils that have antimicrobial properties. Look for products containing essential oils such as tea tree (*Melaleuca alternifolia*), eucalyptus (*Eucalyptus globulus*), lavender (*Lavendula angustifolia*), or orange (*Citrus sinensis*). These concentrated oils kill harmful microorganisms, but they don't contribute to the problem of chemically resistant microbes.

Natural Antiseptic Hand Soap

Buy an unscented liquid hand or body soap and add twenty drops each of lavender, eucalyptus, and orange essential oils to four ounces of the liquid soap. Shake well. Keep a bottle of this fragrant, antiseptic soap in a pump-top dispenser in your kitchen and bathroom for everyday hand washing.

Aromatherapy Room Deodorizer

An aromatherapy spray disinfectant made from essential oils with antimicrobial properties can help to kill airborne microorganisms. Combine eight drops each of lavender and eucalyptus essential oils in a four-ounce glass spray bottle. Fill the bottle with water, shake well, and spritz the air every hour or two, especially if someone in your household is sick. To prevent possible damage, avoid spraying wood surfaces.

Natural Antibacterial Cleanser

To clean hard, nonporous surfaces, such as telephones, countertops, and doorknobs, make a natural antibacterial spray with the following ingredients:

1 tablespoon borax

1 cup hot water

1 cup distilled white vinegar

1/2 teaspoon liquid dishwashing soap

1/2 teaspoon eucalyptus essential oil

1/2 teaspoon lavender essential oil

Combine the borax and hot water and mix thoroughly. Allow to cool to room temperature.

Pour the solution into a spray-top bottle, add the vinegar, dishwashing soap, and essential oils, and shake well.

Just as with most illnesses, the most important thing you can do to prevent colds and flus is to keep yourself as healthy as possible. This means eating a healthful, balanced diet, getting plenty of regular exercise and sufficient sleep, and managing the stressors in your life. When you are vital and enjoying your life, you are much less susceptible to viruses. In the next chapter, you'll learn how your immune system operates to keep you healthy, and you'll discover a number of ways to enhance your immunity.

CHAPTER 2

SIMPLE WAYS TO STRENGTHEN YOUR IMMUNE SYSTEM

Your immune system is the most complex system of your body, and scientists are still uncovering new insights about how the organs, glands, and cells function to maintain health and resist disease. A basic knowledge of how your immune system works will help you better understand how herbs and supplements can support your immune function. Of course, you don't have to understand the intricacies of your immune system for herbs and supplements to be effective!

An Immune System Primer

The immune system is made up of many different components and is spread throughout the body. The thymus gland (found at the base of the neck), spleen (located just under the ribcage on the left side of the body), bone marrow, and a large network of lymph nodes (including the tonsils) make up the basic structure of the immune system. Hundreds of lymph nodes are scattered throughout the body and are concentrated primarily in the armpits, neck, groin, abdomen, and chest.

The thymus gland, spleen, and bone marrow manufacture a variety of infection-fighting white blood cells that circulate throughout the blood and lymph and protect the body from invading microorganisms. In addition, the immune system is composed of specialized cells called macro -

phages and mast cells and special compounds (including interferon, interleukins, and complement fractions) that enhance immune function by stimulating white blood cells to destroy cancer cells and cells infected by microorganisms.

Although it is often ignored, the thymus gland is the most important gland of the immune system and is responsible for a number of immune-related functions. It produces T lymphocytes, white blood cells that are in charge of cell-mediated immunity, and also releases several hormones that regulate immune function. Low levels of thymus hormones are found in the elderly and in people who are under a great deal of stress. If you suffer from frequent or chronic infections, you most likely have impaired thymus function.

The lymphatic system is another critical component of the immune system. Lymph is a clear, colorless fluid that bathes and cleanses all of the cells of your body. It flows through the lymphatic system, a network of porous lymphatic vessels similar to arteries that run parallel to the circulatory system. Lymph passes into and out of the bloodstream through permeable membranes, bringing nutrients to cells and carrying away waste products. Cellular debris is filtered through the lymph nodes, as well as the tonsils, adenoids, appendix, spleen, and Peyer's patches in the small intestine.

Anytime you have an active infection, the lymph nodes closest to the affected area swell to contain the toxins. For example, you've probably noticed tender, swollen lymph nodes under your jaw when you've had a sore throat. As lymph is filtered through the lymph nodes, bacteria and other trouble-causing microorganisms are attacked and consumed by white blood cells. The cells that cleanse the lymph are called macrophages. These large white blood cells, sometimes referred to as "big eaters," engulf and destroy harmful microorganisms, cancer cells, and cellular debris. The lymph nodes also contain B lymphocytes, a type of white blood cell that initiates the production of antibodies in response to infectious microorganisms. When the infection has been overcome, the lymph nodes return to normal, which is about the size of a small pea.

Macrophage
A large white blood cell that devours harmful microorganisms.

Finally, various white blood cells are active participants in your immune system. The primary function of white blood cells is to protect the body against pathogens. Neutrophils play an important role in preventing bacterial infection. They engulf and destroy bacteria, cellular debris, and cancer cells. Lymphocytes are a large family of white blood cells and include T cells, B cells, and natural killer cells. T cells are produced in the thymus gland and circulate throughout the blood and lymph. They are involved in many immune functions, including cell-mediated immunity. There are several different types of T cells, including helper T cells, which support the functioning of other white blood cells; suppressor T cells, which inhibit the activity of other white blood cells; and cytotoxic T cells (also known as killer T cells), which destroy cancer cells and virus-infected cells.

B cells are responsible for producing antibodies to specific antigens, and natural killer cells destroy infected and cancerous cells. Eosinophils and basophils release compounds that break down antigen-antibody complexes and regulate inflammatory and allergic responses. Monocytes are large white blood cells that clean up cellular debris after an infec-

Antigen
A foreign substance, such as a virus, that provokes an immune response.

tion. Macrophages are monocytes that reside in tissues such as the lymph nodes, liver, and spleen.

How Your Immune System Protects You

The primary job of the immune system is to protect the body against infectious microorganisms and to prevent the development of cancer. Your immune system is constantly on patrol, checking cells for evidence of infection and looking for cells that show cancerous changes. The immune system offers two types of protection against disease: nonspecific resistance to disease (also called nonspecific immunity) and specific resistance to disease (also called specific immunity).

Nonspecific immunity
The body's first line of defense against invading microorganisms.

Nonspecific defensive responses are the body's first reaction to invading microorganims, such as the viruses that cause colds and flus. These reactions include the natural barriers provided by healthy skin and mucous membranes, inflammation, fever, and certain antimicrobial chemicals and white blood cells. All nonspecific defenses protect the body against a variety of pathogens and foreign substances. Here's how nonspecific defense works: If infectious microorganisms penetrate the barrier provided by the skin and mucous membranes, antimicrobial chemicals in the blood such as interferons and complement fractions are waiting as a second line of defense. If these fail, the next immune players brought into action include natural killer cells, which kill a wide variety of infectious microorganisms and tumor cells, and phagocytes, white blood cells that engulf and destroy infected and damaged cells.

In addition, inflammation and fever help to

protect the body. When microorganisms invade the body, they damage tissues, causing inflammation (a sore throat is an example of inflammation). Inflammation promotes the disposal of toxins and microorganisms at the site of the injury and prevents the spread of infection. With the extra blood flow that occurs with inflammation, large numbers of white blood cells flood the affected area. They destroy the invaders, and in many cases, this is enough to knock back the infection. Fever also helps the body overcome infection by inhibiting the growth of microbes and enhancing the effect of interferon, the body's natural virus-fighting chemical.

Specific Immunity
The ability of the body to defend itself against specific antigens; also known as immunity.

The second type of protection afforded by the immune system is specific resistance to disease, also known as immunity. This is the ability of the body to defend itself against specific antigens, substances that the immune system recognizes as foreign and that provoke an immune response. There are two types of immune responses involved in specific resistance to disease. These are cell-mediated immune responses and antibody-mediated immune responses.

Cell-mediated immunity begins when T cells (a special type of white blood cell) recognize an antigen (foreign invader). T cells begin a complex process of enlarging, multiplying, and forming highly specialized cells to mount an attack against the invader. This type of immune activity is important for overcoming infection by microorganisms such as viruses, yeast, fungi, parasites, and mold-like bacteria. In addition, cell-mediated immunity protects the body against allergies, autoimmune diseases such as rheumatoid arthritis, and cancer.

In antibody-mediated immune responses, the presence of an antigen stimulates the activation of B cells (specialized types of white blood cells) in the lymph nodes and spleen. They produce plasma cells, which secrete antibodies that travel to the site of the invasion through the lymph and blood. These antibodies combine with the antigen and disable it. Like T cells, specialized B cells remember any antigen that has triggered an immune response and provide long-term immunity to that particular antigen.

How to Keep Your Immune System Healthy

If you're one of those who catch colds easily or come down with more than two colds per year, your immune system is not functioning as well as it could be. Other symptoms of weak immune function include cuts or wounds that are slow to heal; chronic viral, fungal, or yeast infections such as athlete's foot, herpes, or candidiasis; sore or swollen lymph glands; chronic allergies; and any type of recurring infection such as a urinary tract or respiratory infection. Excessive fatigue is another symptom that should alert you to the possibility that your immune system is not functioning up to par.

An overall healthful lifestyle can do much to ensure that your immune system is operating at peak efficiency. Eat a diet of fresh, natural foods, emphasizing organically grown and minimally processed foods. Fresh fruits and vegetables in particular are rich sources of cell-protecting nutrients—strive for at least five, and preferably more, servings daily. Make sure to also get sufficient protein because adequate protein is necessary for making white blood cells and other components of the immune system. Eat two to three servings daily, choosing from fish, lean poultry, eggs, low-fat dairy products, and soy products such as tempeh and tofu.

To prevent immune stress, avoid hydrogenated, polyunsaturated, and saturated fats, and foods treated with chemicals and hormones, all of which create cell damage. Minimize sweets, including honey, maple syrup, and all concentrated sweeteners because all types of sugars have been shown to impair immune function. In addition to maintaining a healthful diet, it's a good idea to take a high-potency multivitamin and mineral supplement. Nutritional deficiencies, especially of the B-complex vitamins and the cell-protecting nutrients A, C, E, selenium, and zinc, are associated with depressed immunity. Finally, avoid tobacco, drugs, and alcohol, all of which inhibit immune function.

Regular daily exercise not only improves your general health, but also specifically strengthens the immune system. But overdoing exercise—more than about an hour a day of aerobic activity—has been shown to actually impair immune function. And emotional stress, as well as physical stress, has a direct negative effect on the immune system. Take time every day to relax and unwind, make sure to get sufficient sleep, and cultivate a positive attitude toward life. In general, happy people are healthier!

If you do come down with a virus, the best approach is to make yourself as comfortable as possible by alleviating the symptoms. As you'll discover in the following chapters on herbs and nutritional supplements, there are specific natural remedies that can lessen the severity of a cold or flu and speed your recovery.

CHAPTER 3

IMMUNE-BOOSTING HERBS: ECHINACEA AND ASTRAGALUS

In addition to supporting your immunity with a healthful lifestyle, there are two herbs that are especially helpful for enhancing your immune function. Astragalus (*Astragalus membranaceous*) is an herb that has been used for centuries in Chinese medicine for bolstering immune function. And echinacea (*Echinacea spp.*) is a native North American plant that has remarkable immune-boosting properties. Both herbs have a specific role in helping to protect you from colds and flus. Astragalus can be taken as a long-term tonic to strengthen immunity; echinacea is excellent for short-term use to provide immediate support to the immune system when a cold or flu threatens. In this chapter, you'll discover everything you need to know to use these herbs effectively.

What Is Echinacea?

Echinacea—pronounced *eck-uh-nay'-sha*—is a member of the compositae family, a large botanical family that includes daisies, marigolds, and dandelions. A one- to four-foot-tall perennial, echinacea is a favorite of gardeners. It looks a lot like black-eyed Susan, with beautiful magenta petals radiating outward from dark cone-shaped centers. (Some less common varieties of echinacea have white or yellow petals.) The name comes from the Greek word *echinos*, meaning sea urchin or hedgehog—an apt description of the prickly cone at the center of the echinacea flower.

Echinacea is native to the plains of the United States, and grows wild nowhere else in the world except for a few places in southern Canada. Of the nine different echinacea species that are indigenous to the United States, three have been used historically and have been clinically studied in both the United States and in Europe: *Echinacea purpurea* (purple coneflower), *Echinacea angustifolia* (narrow-leaved coneflower), and *Echinacea pallida* (pale coneflower). The flower (including seed) and root are the most commonly used parts of the echinacea plant.

How Echinacea Was Discovered

Echinacea has been used for treating colds, coughs, sore throats, and many other types of infectious diseases for centuries. Archeologists have found evidence of echinacea in American Indian sites dating back to the 1600s. Native Americans relied on plants as their primary form of medicine, and echinacea was the favorite herb of the Plains Indians. They used echinacea in a variety of ways: as poultices and teas or they simply chewed on a piece of the root.

Native American tribes generously shared their knowledge of echinacea's healing properties with the European settlers, who quickly adopted the plant. In 1870, Dr. H.C.F. Meyer, a German physician in Pawnee City, Nebraska, concocted a patented herbal medicine made with echinacea. He named it "Meyer's Blood Purifier" and claimed it as a cure-all for a variety of ailments, including snakebite. He believed so strongly in the healing properties of echinacea that in 1887, he tried to promote it to two prominent physicians of the time: Dr. John Uri Lloyd (a professor at the Eclectic Medical Institute in

Cincinnati and later president of the American Pharmaceutical Association) and Dr. John King (author of *King's American Dispensatory*). To prove the efficacy of echinacea, he offered to let himself be bitten by a rattlesnake in the presence of the doctors and to treat himself only with echinacea. The doctors declined his offer, surmising that he was a quack.

Meyer persisted, and persuaded Dr. King to at least give echinacea a try. Although he didn't opt for the snakebite experiment, Dr. King did try echinacea and became convinced of the herb's healing properties. Dr. Lloyd also reversed his previously negative position on echinacea, proclaiming the herb useful for treating many illnesses, including the infectious diseases that were so devastating at that time—diptheria, scarlet fever, influenza, meningitis, measles, and chicken pox.

The Lloyd family pharmaceutical company began marketing echinacea formulations and the herb became extremely popular. At that time, *Echinacea angustifolia* was believed to be the most potent form of the herb. Preparations of echinacea were a common remedy in home medicine chests from the 1890s until the advent of antibiotics in the 1930s. Echinacea and other herbs fell from favor as doctors in the United States began to rely on drugs for treating infectious diseases.

The Reemergence of Echinacea

Fortunately, herbal medicine never took a beating in Europe the way that it did in the United States. European doctors have always regarded herbs as legitimate medical treatments, and herbal products are commonly sold in European pharmacies. Echinacea was introduced to Europe sometime in the early 1900s. In 1932, a German scientist named Gerhard Madaus proved that the fresh-pressed juice from *Echinacea purpurea* flowers had potent immune-strengthening properties. In the ensuing years, approximately 400 scientific studies have proven the powerful, positive effects that echinacea has on the immune system. With these studies, *E. purpurea* became as respected as *E. angustifolia* among herbal practitioners. Since the 1930s, European markets have bought more than 50,000 pounds of echinacea from the United States each year.

Echinacea's long history as a safe infection-fighting herb—in addition to the decades of scientific support that the Europeans have amassed attesting to its efficacy—make echinacea a logical choice for an immune-enhancing herbal medicine.

How Echinacea Protects You

Echinacea protects your body against invading microorganisms in a number of ways. It stimulates the activity of leukocytes, white blood cells that fight infection, and T lymphocytes (also known as killer T cells). It also has action similar to interferon, a protein produced by virus-infected cells that inhibits reproduction of the virus and promotes resistance to further infection. At the same time, echinacea increases the activity of macrophages, white blood cells that engulf and devour harmful microorganisms and infected and damaged cells.

Interferon
A protein produced by virus-infected cells that fights the virus.

In addition to all of the above, echinacea appears to have mild antibiotic properties. And if microbes sneak past your defenses, echinacea can still help. It keeps viruses from gaining a foothold on cell surfaces by blocking virus receptors on cells and prevents microbes from penetrating tissues. It also speeds wound healing by stimulating new, healthy cell growth.

Healing Compounds in Echinacea

Although echinacea is one of the most popular and widely used herbal medicines in the United States and Europe, there is still much to be learned about how it actually works. Researchers differ in their opinions about the most valuable constituents, and to confuse the matter further, different varieties of echinacea contain different constituents. With these considerations in mind, here is a brief attempt to explain the active compounds found in echinacea.

The major important medicinal constituents identified in the plant thus far are polysaccharides, flavonoids, caffeic acid derivatives, essential oils, polyacetylenes, and alkylamides. Many researchers consider polysaccharides to be the primary immune-enhancing ingredient in echinacea. Polysaccharides are large, water-soluble, complex sugar molecules found in plants and mushrooms known to improve immune function.

Polysaccharide
A large, complex sugar molecule found in some plants that stimulates immune function.

Scientists theorize that polysaccharides resem - ble compounds in the cell walls of bacteria and that this case of mistaken identity rouses the immune system into action. But other researchers believe that while the polysaccharides in echinacea do demonstrate strong activity, they may be broken down in the digestive tract before they have a chance to be absorbed into the bloodstream. Echinacea contains a wide variety of immune-enhancing natural chemicals, all of which seem to work together to strengthen immunity.

Echinacoside and cichoric acid are both caffeic acid derivatives and are also water-soluble components of echinacea. Echinacoside is a natural antibiotic and has been used as a marker (a target ingredient) for standardizing some echinacea formulas. But echinacoside has only mild antibiotic activity and has not been shown to actually have immune-enhancing activity. However, in laboratory tests, researchers have found that cichoric acid from echinacea stimulates the activity of macrophages (large white blood cells that gobble up infectious microorganisms).

Other researchers believe that alkylamides and polyacetylenes, the fat-soluble components of echinacea, are primarily responsible for the plant's immune-strengthening benefits. Alkylamides are uncommon plant constituents and give echinacea its unique tongue-tingling sensation. They are found in higher concentrations in *E. purpurea* and *E. angustifolia,* and lower concentrations in *E. pallida.* However, *E. pallida* contains polyacetylenes, which are also considered to have immune-enhancing properties.

It's not unusual that scientists are not united in agreeing on how echinacea works. Isolating the active constituents of a plant is a painstaking process that involves a great deal of research. It's not easy to determine which compounds have medicinal action, and the task is made more difficult because laboratory tests performed on blood samples are not always an accurate reflection of what happens in the body. For example, the medicinal compounds found in plants may work together to create a healing effect and, if they are taken as separate entities, may not have the same effect.

What we do know is that many studies have proven that echinacea improves immune function. Not knowing exactly *how* it strengthens immunity does not negate the positive benefits of this remarkable herb.

Scientific Support for Echinacea

More than 400 scientific studies have proven the effectiveness of echinacea for treating infectious diseases. A 1992 well-designed German research study published in the respected German scientific journal *Zeitschrift fur Phytotherapie* evaluated the effects of echinacea on colds and flu. The double-blind, controlled study involved 180 male and female subjects between eighteen and sixty years of age. (This means that half of the subjects were given an extract of echinacea, and half were given a placebo, and neither group knew if they were receiving echinacea or the placebo.) The researchers found that echinacea both relieved cold and flu symptoms and shortened the duration of the illness. In addition, the researchers discovered that while two droppersful daily of echinacea had some effect, four droppersful daily provided a significant reduction in cold symptoms.

Other studies have reported similar positive results. The Swiss medical journal *Schweizerische Zeitschrift fur Ganzheits Medizin* published a study in 1998 showing that tablets of *Echinacea purpurea* were effective against the common cold. At the University Hospital in Uppsala, Sweden, doctors gave 119 patients echinacea or a placebo, at a dose of two tablets three times a day for eight days. Of the patients taking echinacea, more than three-fourths reported relief from symptoms such as sore throat, fever, nasal congestion, and cough. Echinacea was found to be twice as effective as the placebo in relieving symptoms.

Here's an interesting fact that attests to the popularity and efficacy of echinacea: In 1994 alone, echinacea was prescribed for treating the common cold more than 2.5 million times by German physicians and pharmacists.

How to Use Echinacea for Colds and Flus

Echinacea is commonly used for treating all types of general infections. It is perhaps best known for treating colds and flus and is excellent for other infections such as bronchitis, tonsillitis, strep throat, urinary tract infections, and tooth and gum infections. Echinacea is also useful in helping the immune system knock back fungal infections such as candidiasis.

Infectious diseases respond particularly well to echinacea. This is probably because these diseases are normally dealt with by macrophages and echinacea is especially effective at stimulating macrophage activity.

Taking echinacea to prevent a full-blown cold or flu may be the most effective way to use it. Nipping any infection in the bud is the most assured way of avoiding a more serious illness, so it's always a good idea to take echinacea at the very first indication of a cold or flu, such as a scratchy throat, runny nose, or sneezing. At the first sign of symptoms, take one dropperful of extract or two capsules or tablets four times a day and continue until symptoms are relieved, or up to ten days.

A number of laboratory studies have been performed on echinacea using many times the therapeutic dose given to humans, with no toxic side effects. However, the German Commission E, the German authority on herbal remedies, cautions that echinacea should not be used by people who are susceptible to allergic reactions, especially to the compositae (daisy) family. To err on the side of caution, if you have never taken echinacea, begin with a low dose for a couple of days to rule out any individual sensitivity to the herb. For example, try taking ten drops of echinacea liquid extract two times a day and gradually increase the dosage until you are taking the full amount, generally recommended as one dropperful (approximately one-half teaspoon) three times a day.

The most common side effect that can occur with echinacea is caused by taking liquid echinacea extract. Some people report a burning sensation in the back of the throat when they take undiluted echinacea. Others experience a transient tingling sensation on the tongue or a feeling of nausea associated with the increased salivation that echinacea causes. While unpleasant, none of these symptoms are harmful, and all can be avoided by diluting echinacea extract in a small amount of warm water or by taking echinacea in capsules or tablets.

Choosing an Echinacea Product

All parts of the echinacea plant—the flowers (which contain the seed heads), leaves, stems, and roots—have medicinal properties, although the roots and seeds are considered to have the most powerful benefits. In addition, all varieties of echinacea appear to have immune-enhancing properties, although they differ in their chemical makeup. The varieties of echinacea commonly used in commercial echinacea preparations are *Echinacea purpurea, Echinacea angustifolia,* and *Echinacea pallida.*

The aerial parts of the plant (the flower heads, leaves, and stems) are harvested when the plant is blooming, generally in the late summer. The roots are harvested in the late fall from plants that are three to four years old. Many herbalists and herbal manufacturers agree that echinacea products should contain at least one part of or a combination of the root, leaf, and flower of *E. purpurea* plus the root of *E. angustifolia.* While *E. pallida* is sometimes included in echinacea preparations, it has not been studied as extensively as *E. purpurea* or *E. angustifolia*.

The majority of scientific and clinical studies on echinacea have used a German product made from the freshly pressed juice of *E. purpurea's* flowering plant tops stabilized with alcohol (this preparation is known as a "succus"). This does not mean that other types of echinacea preparations are not just as valuable. There are many different types of echinacea products on the market, including liquid extracts made with grain alcohol or glycerin and water; capsules or tablets of freeze-dried extracts or simple herb powders; and *E. purpurea* succus.

A simple guideline is to remember that an herbal preparation can only be as potent as the raw plant material that goes into it. The fresher the plant, the more likely it is to contain a high concentration of active ingredients. Therefore, when buying echinacea products, look for those made from fresh plants. Read product labels—they will clearly state if fresh echinacea was used.

What Is Astragalus?

Astragalus (*Astragalus membranaceous*) is a member of the legume family and is a close relative of peas and licorice. Native to northern China and Mongolia, astragalus is a perennial, straggly plant that grows up to two feet tall and has small yellow flowers and one-inch pea-like pods. However, it's the taproot that contains the healing properties. The thick, multibranched, dark-brown root has a creamy-yellow interior and a slightly sweet, celery-like flavor. This mild, pleasant-tasting herb is one of the most potent immune-strengthening herbs known.

Astragalus has been used for at least 2,000 years in China and continues to be one of the most frequently prescribed herbal medicines in

Chinese medicine. The first recorded mention of astragalus was in an ancient Chinese medical text, *The Divine Husbandman's Classic of the Materia Medica.* For centuries, astragalus has been prescribed by practitioners of traditional Chinese medicine to strengthen overall vitality, which the Chinese refer to as *qi.* In fact, the name for astragalus in Chinese is huang qi, or yellow energy.

In Chinese medicine, astragalus is viewed as a general strengthening herb and is included in many immune-supportive formulas. It is regarded as beneficial for the entire body and is considered to have effects similar to ginseng, although milder and therefore safer for general use. For thousands of years, astragalus has been used for treating general fatigue, frequent colds, poor digestion, chronic lung weakness, diabetes, and heart disease, and to protect the liver against toxins. In hospitals in China, astragalus is used to help people who are undergoing chemotherapy to regain healthy immune function.

Although bacteria and viruses were unknown to the ancient Chinese and they didn't have the knowledge of the immune system that we have today, they theorized that astragalus increased the protective energy that shielded the body from invasion by "vicious energies." Recent scientific research is proving that although the language may be different, the concept that astragalus protects the body against disease is accurate.

How Astragalus Works

Astragalus is most commonly used as a general tonic for improving health and specifically for enhancing immune function. Because of its ability to safely strengthen immunity, astragalus is an excellent herbal tonic that can be taken on a regular basis for helping the body ward off colds and flus. Not only does astragalus stimulate immune activity, but it also has the remarkable ability to help restore healthy functioning to a suppressed immune system.

Scientific studies have proven that astragalus contains active compounds that stimulate the immune system. Scientists are still figuring out exactly how astragalus works, but research indicates that it is likely the polysaccharides (astragalan I, II, and III) and the saponins (astramembrannin I and II) in the herb that are responsible for bolstering immune function. What scientists have found is that astragalus strengthens two important aspects of immunity: nonspecific immunity, which defends the body against invading microorganisms, and specific immunity, which uses specific antibodies against specific invaders or antigens.

There are several ways in which astragalus enhances nonspecific immunity: it stimulates the production of interferon, which inhibits the ability of viruses to reproduce; it increases the number of natural killer cells, which seek out and destroy cells that are infected by viruses and cancer; and it steps up the production of macrophages.

Natural Killer Cell
A type of white blood cell that kills infectious micro-organisms.

Astragalus improves specific immunity by increasing levels of various antibodies, also called immunoglobulins. For example, studies have shown that astragalus increases levels of immune-enhancing immunoglobulin A (IgA) and immunoglobulin G (IgG). IgA keeps invading microorganisms from setting up housekeeping in the mucous membranes of the respiratory tract and other areas of the body, while IgG is the primary antibody that circulates in the bloodstream. In another study, astragalus was shown to increase levels of immunoglobulin E (IgE) and immunoglobulin M (IgM). IgE is important for easing inflammation and allergic responses, and IgM helps to activate a special protein called complement fraction, which supports antibodies in fighting bacteria and other harmful micro-organisms.

Scientific Support for Astragalus

Numerous scientific studies support the traditional use of astragalus as a tonic for improving general health and as a specific enhancer of immune function. Many of the studies have been conducted in China, where astragalus has had a long history of use.

Much research has been done regarding the use of astragalus for treating colds and other upper respiratory infections. In one study of 1,000 people with lowered immunity, astragalus was clearly beneficial. Over a two-month period, subjects were given astragalus; as a result, they experienced fewer colds, and if they did become sick, their colds were less severe and of shorter duration. Researchers found that astragalus increased levels of immunoglobulin A (IgA) and immuno-globulin G (IgG), both of which play important roles in fighting off cold and flu viruses.

In a study involving twenty-eight people, those who were given an extract of astragalus for two months were found to have significantly higher levels of interferon compared with those who were not given the herb. Interferon interferes with the ability of viruses, such as the microorganisms that cause colds and flu, to replicate.

In a study at the University of Texas Medical Center in Houston, a team of Chinese and American researchers studied the effects of astragalus on immune cells taken from people with cancer. The researchers found that astragalus stimulated an increase in the functioning of T cells, which are an important part of the immune system's surveillance and essential to the body's ability to overcome viruses.

How to Use Astragalus

In traditional Chinese medicine, astragalus is classified as a warming herb and therefore is not used during an acute illness that has symptoms of fever (such as a cold or flu) because it can exacerbate symptoms. However, astragalus is excellent for bolstering the immune system and helping to prevent colds and flus. To enhance immunity, take astragalus throughout the cold and flu season, or for at least one month in the early fall to build immune strength for the winter.

Astragalus is sold in a variety of forms including capsules and liquid extracts. Take two 500-mg capsules of dried powdered root three times daily, or one-half to one teaspoon of the liquid extract twice daily. The dried root is also available either shredded or in long, thin, flat slices that look something like tongue depressors. In China, slices of astragalus are made into teas or added to soups and other dishes.

To make a strong astragalus tea in the traditional Chinese method, simmer two ounces of dried astragalus root in approximately two and one-half cups of water in a covered pot for one hour. Strain, saving the liquid, and cook the herb a second time by simmering in one and one-half cups of water for thirty minutes. Strain, and combine the liquid from the first cooking with the liquid from the second. Drink one cup of this tea in the morning and another in the evening, fifteen minutes before meals. Astragalus has a sweet, pleasant flavor. Refrigerate leftover tea for up to two days and warm it gently before drinking.

Immune-Building Herbal Tonic Soup

A savory vegetable soup is a traditional way of incorporating astragalus into your diet. Eat this soup at least twice a week during the fall and winter to boost immunity. Astragalus root is tough and inedible, so you'll need to remove the root slices before eating the soup.

1 ounce sliced dried astragalus root

1-inch piece fresh ginger root, slivered

¼ cup uncooked brown basmati rice

8 cups vegetable or chicken stock

2 tablespoons olive oil

1 cup chopped onion

1 cup diced carrots

½ cup sliced shiitake mushrooms

6 cloves garlic, minced

2 tablespoons light miso, or to taste

¼ cup minced parsley

Simmer the astragalus, ginger, rice, and stock in a heavy, covered pot for one hour. Sauté the onions, carrots, and shiitake mushrooms in olive oil for five minutes. Add the garlic and sauté for one minute.

Add the sautéed vegetable mixture to the soup pot, cover, and simmer for thirty minutes. Remove the astragalus.

Dilute the miso in a small amount of hot broth and add to soup. Add parsley, let stand for five minutes, and serve.

CHAPTER 4

VIRUS-FIGHTING HERBS: ELDERBERRY AND GARLIC

Elderberry (*Sambucus nigra*) and garlic (*Allium sativum*) are two herbs that are essential for helping to fight the viruses that cause colds and flus. Both can be taken regularly throughout cold and flu season to help ward off viruses. In the event that a virus does sneak past your immune defenses, both elderberry and garlic can help to rally your immune system to effectively fight off the trouble-causing microorganisms. In this chapter, you'll learn how these herbs work to defend you and how to best use them.

What Is Elderberry?

Elder is a small, flowering shrub or small tree native to Europe and North Africa and naturalized throughout the United States. The fruits (or berries) have long been used as a food, with some of the most popular uses being wine, jam, and pie.

Medicinally, elderberries have been used for at least 2,500 years as a folk remedy for the treatment of colds, flu, and upper respiratory infections. In ancient times, elder was regarded as a sacred tree in mythology and folklore. Elder trees were believed to offer protection against evil influences and were planted near English cottages for this reason. Modern science is finding that black elderberry does possess protective powers against certain "evil influences"—specifically, the viruses that cause influenza.

Prescribed medicinally since the time of Hippocrates, the beautiful, white, fragrant flowers are traditionally made into a tea to ease fevers (you'll find a recipe for elderflower tea in Chapter 7). But it's the dark purple berries that hold the most promise as a remedy for colds and flus. When taken throughout cold and flu season or even at the first sign of a viral infection, elderberries have the unique ability to stop a virus in its tracks.

How Elderberry Works

Scientific studies in recent years have demonstrated the powerful virus-fighting properties of elderberries. In fact, an extract of elderberry has been shown to be effective against all strains of influenza virus. Here's how the herb works.

Viruses aren't able to reproduce on their own, but need living cells to replicate themselves. Virus cells are covered with tiny spikes called hemagglutinin. They take over cells by puncturing the cell walls with these spikes. These spikes are coated with an enzyme called neuraminidase, which aids in breaking down the cell walls. But elderberry has the ability to inhibit the activity of neuraminidase and to disarm the spikes, thereby thwarting the flu viruses and keeping them from invading cells. Scientists have found two active ingredients in elderberry that disarm neuraminidase within twenty-four to forty-eight hours of taking the herb.

Neuraminidase
An enzyme used by viruses to break down healthy cell walls.

Scientific Support for Elderberry

Since the 1980s, the Israeli virologist Madeleine Mumcuoglu (mum-shu-glu) of the Hadassah University Medical Center in Jerusalem has studied the antiviral properties of black elderberry for treating colds, flus, and respiratory infections. Most of her work has been in the laboratory, where she and her colleagues have isolated the active ingredients in elderberry and tested them on viruses. In her research, she discovered two active principles that effectively disarmed the flu virus. Mumcuoglu found that compounds in elderberrry bind to the spikes on the surface of virus cells and prevent them from puncturing cell membranes. In addition, the high concentrations of bioflavonoids in elderberry inhibit the action of neuraminidase. She tested her proprietary extract of elderberry (Sambucol) against various strains of influenza A and B in the laboratory and found the herb effective against all types of flu.

Bioflavonoid
A nutrient that strengthens capillary walls.

In 1993 a flu epidemic at an Israeli Kibbutz provided the opportunity to test elderberry on patients. In people presenting with full-blown flu symptoms, half of the subjects were given four tablespoons of standardized elderberry extract daily, and the other half were given a placebo. Within twenty-four hours, 20 percent of the patients receiving elderberry showed a dramatic reduction in flu symptoms such as fever, cough, and muscle pain. Within forty-eight hours, 75 percent were greatly improved, and within seventy-two hours, 90 percent had completely recovered from the flu. In contrast, only 8 percent of those taking the placebo began to improve after twenty-four hours; the remaining 92 percent took six days to improve. The results were reported in the Winter 1995 issue of *The Journal of Alternative and Complementary Medicine*.

How to Use Elderberry

Many types of elderberry products are available at natural foods stores and pharmacies. While research studies have focused on the proprietary extract Sambucol, it's likely that other extracts of elderberry are also effective.

To prevent colds and flus, take one-half teaspoon of liquid extract or one to two teaspoons of elderberry syrup twice daily throughout cold and flu season. If you come down with the symptoms of a cold or flu, increase your dosage to one teaspoon of extract or one tablespoon of syrup four times a day.

You can use dried elderberries to make your own liquid extract and syrup. Buy the elderberries at an herb store or natural foods store. To make elderberry extract, fill a wide-mouth glass canning jar two-thirds full of the berries and add enough vodka to fill the jar. Stir well, cover, and let the berries steep for three weeks, giving the jar a good shake once a day. Strain the extract through several layers of cheesecloth, squeezing as much liquid as possible out of the berries. Store the extract in a glass bottle in a cool, dark place.

To make elderberry syrup, pour four cups of boiling water over two cups of dried elderberries. Soak for eight hours, and then simmer, covered, for thirty minutes. Strain, measure the remaining liquid, and add an equal amount of honey to the liquid (discard the berries). Gently reheat the mixture until the honey has completely dissolved. Pour into a clean glass bottle and store in the refrigerator.

Elderberry occasionally causes stomach upset, including abdominal cramps or diarrhea. If this occurs, take it with meals.

Garlic: More Than a Kitchen Herb

Garlic (*Allium sativum*) is probably the best known and most beloved herb in the world. Not only does the pungent bulb have a prominent place in most cuisines, but it is also one of the world's oldest medicines, and remains as useful today as it was in ancient times.

A member of the lily family, garlic is a close relative of onions, scallions, chives, and shallots. Botanists believe that garlic probably originated in central Asia, but the plant has been cultivated for centuries around the world. More than 700 species of garlic are found today in North America, Europe, Asia, and North Africa.

Although all parts of the garlic plant are edible, the bulb of the plant is what is used in medicine and as a food (although young garlic greens are sometimes used in cooking). The English name "garlic" is derived from the ancient Anglo-Saxon words "gar," which means spear, and "lac," the word for plant; referring to the long, thin, spear-shaped leaves. The genus name *Allium* most likely comes from a Celtic word that means burning (as in sensation), which garlic certainly does produce when eaten raw.

Our Ambivalent Love of Garlic

There's no question that garlic has been revered for centuries—the first known prescription for garlic was chiseled onto a Sumerian clay tablet in about 3000 B.C. Garlic was a favorite remedy of the ancient Egyptians, who believed the herb increased endurance and prevented illness. They fed vast quantities of garlic to the workers who built the great pyramids, in hopes of keeping them healthy and strong.

Greek and Roman physicians also valued garlic and recommended it for treating colds, infections, wounds, cancer, and heart problems. In ancient India, garlic was used to treat colds, leprosy, and heart disease, while doctors in China prescribed garlic for respiratory infections, intestinal parasites, and skin problems. All of these prescriptions for garlic, first made thousands of years ago, are supported today by scientific research.

Long before the discovery of viruses and bacteria, people recognized that garlic offered protection against infectious diseases. During the Middle Ages, garlic was used by some to ward off the bubonic plague. And prior to the discovery of penicillin in 1928, garlic was the treatment of choice for infections such as pneumonia, bronchitis, tuberculosis, and dysentery.

Throughout history, though, there have been many people who have shunned garlic because of its pungent odor. In ancient Rome and Greece, many upper-class citizens associated garlic with the lower classes, and the wealthy in medieval Europe considered the consumption of garlic to be fitting only for those of low social status. In seventeenth-century England, garlic was eaten with gusto by the peasants, but used only sparingly by the upper classes, even though they recognized the usefulness of the herb for treating many infectious illnesses. In nineteenth-century America, the same ambivalence about garlic continued. While the herb was believed to be effective for treating colds and other respiratory ailments, many found the smell offensive.

Despite our ambivalence about garlic, the herb is more popular now than ever. Not only is it a staple in most kitchens, but enthusiasm for the health-protective benefits of garlic have made garlic supplements one of the top-selling herbal products in the United States.

How Garlic Works

Most of the health benefits of garlic are attributed to its sulfur compounds, of which there are more than 100. While researchers are still exploring exactly which compounds are responsible for the wide range of garlic's therapeutic effects, studies indicate that the compound alliin (al-lee-in) appears to be the primary source of the herb's antimicrobial properties. Alliin is responsible for the characteristic pungent odor and taste of garlic.

When chopped, crushed, or chewed, alliin comes into contact with another garlic compound, the enzyme allinase, and **Allicin** is transformed into allicin, a powerful antibiotic that is effective *A powerful anti-* against a wide variety of bacteria, *biotic compound* ria, viruses, and fungi. In fact, one *created when garlic* medium clove of raw garlic is *is crushed, chewed,* estimated to have the same anti-*or chopped.* bacterial effect as 100,000 units of penicillin. (An oral dose of penicillin ranges from 600,000 to 1.2 million units, which equals six to twelve cloves of garlic.) Allicin is also the precursor to other healing compounds in garlic, including ajoene, diallyl sufide, and other sulfur-containing complexes.

In addition to sulfur compounds, garlic also contains amino acids, glycosides, vitamins A, B, C, and E, and the trace minerals germanium and selenium. Germanium is an immune enhancer that helps the body eliminate toxic metals, and selenium is a powerful antioxidant that supports the immune system.

Scientific Support for Garlic

Scientists are proving what the ancient Egyptians knew centuries ago—garlic is a potent ally in helping to fight cold and flu viruses. In a recent study reported in *Advances in Therapy*, Peter Jossling of the Garlic Centre in East Sussex, England, found that a daily garlic supplement cut the incidence of colds in half. The researchers also discovered that study participants who did get sick recovered more quickly than did those not taking garlic.

In the study, 146 volunteers were randomly assigned to two groups. One group received a garlic supplement containing allicin, the ingredient in garlic that has been identified as having antimicrobial properties. The other group was given a placebo. Over a twelve-week period between November and February, the volunteers were required to keep a daily diary in which they recorded any cold symptoms and rated their health using a five-point scale.

At the end of the study, researchers found that the group given the garlic supplement reported twenty-four colds, as compared with the placebo group, which reported sixty-five colds. The people who were given the placebo also reported more than three times as many days that they were "challenged virally" (366 for the placebo group as opposed to 111 for the group taking garlic), and those taking the placebo also reported suffering symptoms for a lengthier period than did those taking garlic.

How to Use Fresh Garlic

Garlic is available in a variety of forms including capsules, tablets, extracts, and gel capsules. And, of course, there's always the real thing—fresh garlic. Eating just one clove of garlic a day can help to ward off the microorganisms that cause colds and flus as well as improve overall health.

Fresh garlic is available year-round in the United States. The primary types available are the white-skinned, pungent California variety and the milder-flavored purple-skinned Mexican and Italian type. Both varieties contain the desirable immune-enhancing compounds. Elephant garlic, which looks like giant garlic, is actually a form of leek. It has a much milder flavor than does garlic and doesn't offer the same degree of health-enhancing properties as true garlic does.

When buying garlic, choose plump, solid bulbs, and avoid those with soft spots. The bulbs should be heavy; if they feel light, the garlic cloves are too dry. Look for bulbs with large individual cloves, because they're easier to peel. To keep garlic cloves from sprouting, store them in a cool, dark place, but not in the refrigerator.

Cooking and Eating Fresh Garlic

To peel a clove of garlic, place it on a cutting board and lay the flat side of a broad knife on top. With your free hand, gently hit the side of the blade with your fist or the heel of your hand. This will crack the skin that covers the clove, and you can then easily peel the clove.

Because raw garlic is so pungent, not many people enjoy simply chewing on a plain, raw clove of garlic. In fact, consuming raw garlic in this way can cause mouth irritation, nausea, and stomach upset. Instead, add finely minced garlic to salad dressings, baked potatoes, or cottage cheese. You can also sprinkle chopped raw garlic on pasta dishes or soups just before serving.

Although raw garlic contains the highest concentration of antibiotic properties, lightly cooked garlic does retain some health benefits. If you're going to cook garlic, just be sure to let it stand for ten minutes after chopping it. This allows the antibiotic compound allicin to fully develop. And whenever possible, add garlic at the end of the cooking time—preferably during the last five minutes—of the dish you're preparing.

To subdue the pungency of raw garlic, try making marinated garlic. Peel garlic cloves and fill a glass jar two-thirds full of the garlic. Combine equal parts of balsamic vinegar, soy sauce, and honey and heat gently until the honey liquifies. Pour over the garlic cloves, making sure that the liquid covers the garlic by at least one inch.

Let cool to room temperature and cover the jar with a lid. Place in the refrigerator for a couple of weeks before eating. Marinated garlic is delicious eaten as a snack and can be added to salad dressings, soups, stir-fried rice, or vegetables. Once opened, it will keep for at least one month in the refrigerator.

There's no question that garlic causes garlic breath, which can last for several hours after you have eaten it. If the odor bothers you (or others!), try chewing a sprig of parsley or a few fennel seeds to neutralize the odor.

How to Use Garlic Supplements

If you don't like fresh garlic, you can always turn to garlic supplements. Garlic supplements vary widely in their potency, but in general, you should take between 600 and 900 mg per day of powdered garlic in capsules or tablets; 4 ml per day of aged garlic liquid extract; or 10 mg per day of garlic oil gel capsules. These amounts provide the equivalent dosage of one medium-size clove of fresh garlic.

For best effect, garlic should be eaten daily. In addition to its antibiotic properties, garlic has natural anticlotting properties, which make it helpful for preventing strokes and heart attacks. However, if you are taking prescription anti-coagulants, you should check with your doctor before taking garlic supplements or eating raw garlic daily.

CHAPTER 5

VIRUS-FIGHTING NUTRIENTS: VITAMIN C, N-ACETYLCYSTEINE, AND ZINC

In addition to boosting your immune system and fighting off viruses, specific nutrients play an important role in your efforts to resist colds and flus. Vitamin C, N-acetylcysteine, and zinc are three nutrients you should know about. In this chapter, you'll learn how these nutrients help to protect you, and how to use them effectively.

Why Vitamin C Is Essential

Vitamin C bathes every cell of the body and plays a key role in many vital bodily functions, including the health of the immune system. The scientific name, ascorbic acid, means "without scurvy," referring to the disease caused by a deficiency of this essential vitamin. Scurvy is characterized by hemorraging of capillaries in the skin and weakening of bone and cartilage and is always fatal if left untreated. This painful disease often afflicted sailors on long voyages, who subsisted primarily on grains while at sea. In the mid-eighteenth century, vitamins had not yet been discovered, but people realized that eating fresh fruits and vegetables prevented scurvy. British sailors began taking along rations of limes, hence they became commonly known as "limeys." In 1917, the specific protective substance in fruits and vegetables was identified as vitamin C.

Since that time, a great deal of research has investigated the role of vitamin C in health. Vitamin C is essential for the formation of collagen, a protein necessary for the development of skin, bones, tendons, and connective tissues. It protects the cardiovascular system by lowering blood pressure and improving the flexibility of blood vessels, reduces the risk of stroke, has powerful antioxidant properties that help to prevent the development of cancer, and enhances immune function.

How Vitamin C Protects Against Colds

Vitamin C first became noted as a cold remedy in 1970, when Linus Pauling, Ph.D, published *Vitamin C and the Common Cold.* Pauling, an esteemed two-time Nobel laureate scientist, maintained that high doses of vitamin C could protect against colds. Dozens of research studies in the ensuing three decades have shown that although vitamin C probably won't keep you from catching a cold, it can lessen the symptoms if you take a large amount (1,000 mg or more) at the first sign of infection.

Vitamin C works in several ways to improve the body's ability to overcome a virus. It stimulates the release of interferon, a protein substance that helps the body resist viruses. It also enhances the activity of phagocytes, white blood cells that kill viruses. The powerful antioxidant activity of vitamin C helps to protect the immune system from damage by viruses. And vitamin C has natural antihistamine action, which helps reduce congestion.

Antihistamine
A substance that blocks histamine, which causes the symptoms of allergies such as congestion.

Interestingly, almost all animals synthesize vitamin C from glucose (blood sugar), but humans do not. Scientists believe that a gene necessary for the production of vitamin C was somehow damaged about 35 million years ago in our ancestors, making it necessary for us to obtain the vitamin through dietary sources.

The current recommended amount of vitamin C suggested by the government is 75 mg daily for women and 90 mg for men. This amount can easily be obtained by eating citrus fruits, cantaloupe, broccoli, bell peppers, tomatoes, and dark-green leafy vegetables, but few people actually eat enough of these foods on a daily basis to acquire sufficient levels of vitamin C. In fact, various studies show that three-quarters or more of Americans don't consume five servings of fruits and vegetables daily, the minimum amount recommended for health. And to obtain the larger amounts that appear to be most effective for preventing and treating colds and flus, supplements are generally necessary.

Scientific Support for Vitamin C

In a 2002 study published in the journal *Advances in Therapy*, researchers tracked the incidence of colds in 168 volunteers for two months. The volunteers were split into two groups; half received supplements of vitamin C and the other half received a placebo. Researchers found that those taking vitamin C had significantly fewer colds (37 versus 50 in the control group), less severe symptoms, and a quicker recovery.

A study in the October 1999 issue of the *Journal of Manipulative and Physiological Therapeutics* evaluated the efficacy of large doses of vitamin C in preventing and relieving cold and flu symptoms. In the study, 715 students between the ages of eighteen and thirty-two were divided into two groups. Those in the control group (consisting of 463 students) were given pain relievers and decongestants when they presented with cold or flu symptoms. Those in the test group (consisting of 252 students) were treated with vitamin C when they presented with cold or flu symptoms; 1,000 mg hourly for the first six hours, and then three times daily thereafter. (Those students in the test group who did not have symptoms were also given 1,000 mg of vitamin C three times daily during the study.) The researchers found that cold and flu symptoms of those treated with vitamin C decreased by 85 percent as compared to the control group.

How to Use Vitamin C

To keep your immune system healthy, it's a good idea to take a supplement of at least 250 mg of vitamin C daily. But you should still eat at least five servings of fresh fruits and vegetables every day. Fresh fruits and vegetables contain numerous beneficial compounds that have health-protective benefits that no supplement can match.

To use vitamin C for treating a cold or flu, take up to 5,000 mg daily at the first sign of symptoms—a scratchy throat, sneezing, or a runny nose. It's best to divide up the dosage, taking 500 mg every hour or two to maintain constant levels of vitamin C in the bloodstream. Because vitamin C is nontoxic and water-soluble, any excess that is not utilized by the body is easily excreted by the kidneys.

Large amounts of vitamin C can sometimes cause gastrointestinal distress such as cramping, diarrhea, and nausea. These symptoms generally disappear with the use of a buffered form of vitamin C. It's also best to divide your intake of vitamin C into two or more doses throughout the day, which improves absorption and decreases the likelihood of gastrointestinal distress. During times of stress or illness, the body's need for vitamin C increases, and tolerance for the vitamin also tends to increase.

N-acetylcysteine (NAC): A Promising Cold and Flu Remedy

You may never have heard of this nutrient, but N-acetylcysteine (commonly called NAC) is an immune-boosting supplement that can help to increase your resistance to colds and flus. NAC is a form of the amino acid cysteine, and is naturally produced by the body. It helps the liver neutralize toxic compounds and encourages the production of the enzyme glutathione, one of the body's most potent antioxidants. By boosting glutathione production, NAC supports the immune system's defenses against viruses and other invading microorganisms.

Glutathione
A powerful antioxidant made by the body and found in some foods, including asparagus and avocados.

Since the 1960s, NAC has been used to help dissolve the thick mucus that clogs the lungs of people suffering from chronic respiratory ailments such as bronchitis, sinusitis, asthma, and pneumonia. Because of NAC's ability to increase gluta-thione and clear mucous congestion, researchers have tested the nutrient to determine its effectiveness in preventing and relieving cold and flu symptoms.

Scientific Support for NAC

In a study reported in the *European Respiratory Journal,* Silvio De Flora, M.D., found that taking NAC significantly decreased the incidence of flu symptoms, even in people who had been infected with a flu virus. In the study, 262 subjects at the University of Genoa, Italy were given either two 600-mg tablets of NAC or two placebos daily for six months throughout the flu season. The participants were required to keep a daily log of their health and any flu symptoms, and some were tested for flu antibodies.

Of those who had laboratory-confirmed cases of the flu, only 25 percent of those taking NAC developed symptoms. However, 79 percent of those taking the placebo developed flu symptoms. Those taking NAC also reported less severe symptoms and recovered more quickly than those taking the placebo. "An additional criterion for evaluating the severity of influenza-like episodes was the length of time in bed, which, irrespective of the age of patients, was remarkably shorter in NAC-treated subjects," noted Dr. De Flora.

Because not everyone who gets sick comes down with a full-blown case of the flu, Dr. De Flora and his associates also evaluated the effects of NAC on more general flu-like symptoms, such as nasal discharge, sore throat, achiness, headache, fever, and cough. They found that the people who were taking NAC had only one-third to one-half of the flu-like symptoms of those who were taking the placebo.

During the study, general immune function was periodically tested in all of the subjects. In the tests, antigens (noninfectious bacterial compounds) that trigger an immune response were applied to the skin. The elderly people in the study had a noticeably sluggish immune response to these antigens, which indicates decreased immune function. However, for those taking NAC, immune responsiveness steadily improved over the course of the study—but not for those taking the placebo.

Dr. De Flora concluded that NAC could provide broad-spectrum protection to prevent, or at least minimize, the symptoms of infection and could be especially helpful for the elderly and other people at risk for contracting the flu.

How to Use NAC

If you want to try NAC for flu prevention, take a

500-mg tablet once daily. It is most effective when taken on an empty stomach. If you come down with flu symptoms, take 500–1,000 mg three times a day, or up to 3,000 mg a day. Because NAC can increase the excretion of copper in the urine, it's a good idea to add a mineral supplement that includes copper (2 mg daily) and zinc (30 mg daily) if you are taking NAC for more than a couple of weeks.

NAC is considered safe and nontoxic, and has no side effects when taken at the recommended dosage. However, exceeding the dosage may cause gastrointestinal distress. Because there are no studies of NAC in pregnant women, it's not recommended for women who are pregnant.

How Zinc Enhances Immunity

Zinc is an important trace mineral needed for the proper functioning of the immune system. It's found in a wide variety of foods, including oysters (the richest source of zinc), meat, seafood, eggs, seeds, nuts, and whole grains. But the average daily diet often falls far short of the minimum amount needed for health, and there are many factors that interfere with obtaining adequate zinc. For example, if you eat less than about 2,400 calories a day or if you gravitate toward a vegetarian diet (or simply avoid red meat), you are probably lacking in zinc. Even a high-fiber diet, which is generally recognized as a healthful habit, can interfere with zinc absorption.

Zinc affects immune function in several ways. It helps to maintain the health of the thymus gland, which tends to shrink with age. The thymus plays a critical role in immune function and acts directly against certain viruses that cause the common cold. Zinc also plays an essential role in maintaining the health of the immune system. When zinc levels are insufficient, the number of

T cells drops, certain infection-fighting white blood cells are compromised, and thymus hormone levels decrease.

Scientific Support for Zinc

In a double-blind clinical trial, researchers found that zinc lozenges significantly reduced the duration of the common cold. As reported in the 1996 issue of *Annals of Internal Medicine*, physicians at the Cleveland Clinic divided clinic employees into two groups. Forty-nine people were given lozenges containing 13.3 mg of zinc gluconate-glycine, and fifty received placebo lozenges. Each participant joined the study within twenty-four hours of developing cold symptoms and was instructed to take one lozenge every two waking hours.

The researchers found that the people who were taking the zinc lozenges had cold symptoms an average of 4.4 days, as compared to 7.6 days for those taking the placebo lozenges. In addition, those taking the zinc lozenges had fewer days with sore throat, nasal congestion and drainage, headache, coughing, and hoarseness. The symptoms of fever, muscle aches, and sneezing were almost the same for both groups.

"Our study showed that the time to resolution of all symptoms was significantly shorter in the zinc group," wrote lead investigator Michael L. Macknin, M.D. The researchers theorize that zinc prevents the replication of the cold virus and stabilizes cell membranes. In addition, zinc may enhance the production of interferon, the body's natural antiviral substance.

How to Use Zinc

It's best to start taking zinc lozenges immediately when you notice the first symptoms of a cold or flu, within twenty-four hours of the symptoms' appearance. Avoid buying zinc lozenges that contain sorbitol, mannitol, or citric acid, because these substances bind with zinc and make it less effective. Instead, buy tablets that are sweetened with glycine (an amino acid). The lozenges should contain between 15 and 25 mg of zinc gluconate, which appears to be one of the most absorbable forms.

At the first appearance of cold or flu symptoms, take two lozenges, followed by one lozenge every two hours that you are awake for the first two days, for a maximum of about 150 mg of zinc daily. On the third day, cut the dosage in half and continue for up to seven days if necessary. It's important to allow the lozenges to dissolve slowly in your mouth because it's necessary for zinc to come into direct contact with the mouth and throat tissues in order to disarm the virus.

Zinc may cause an unpleasant aftertaste that can linger, affecting the flavor of any foods or beverages consumed for several hours. Zinc lozenges also can cause mouth irritation and nausea for some people. Because too much zinc can actually lower immune function, you shouldn't take high doses of zinc for more than a week at a time. However, some zinc is necessary for a healthy immune system, and it's a good idea to take a multivitamin and mineral supplement that supplies between 15 and 25 mg of zinc daily.

CHAPTER 6

WHY YOU SHOULDN'T TAKE DRUGS FOR COLDS AND FLUS

The shelves of pharmacies and grocery stores are lined with dozens of remedies to ease the symptoms of colds and flus. Chances are, you have at least a few such remedies in your household medicine chest. But pain and fever relievers, cough medicines, decongestants, and other medications interfere with your body's attempt at healing and can cause a cold or flu to linger. In addition, many over-the-counter cold and flu medicines can have unpleasant and even dangerous side effects.

Drugs You Should Avoid and Why

In a 1990 study reported in the *Journal of Infectious Diseases,* researchers found that people who took aspirin and acetaminophen for cold and flu symptoms suppressed their immune system's ability to destroy the cold virus. In general, it's best to avoid these medicines if possible. In most cases, you can successfully lower a fever using natural remedies such as yarrow and elderflower tea and cool sponge baths (see Chapter 7 for remedies).

A runny nose almost always occurs with a cold or flu, especially in the initial stages. Many people turn to antihistamines to dry up excess mucus, but these medications often have the effect of making you sleepy. Worse, they can increase the risk of a sinus infection because they thicken mucus, which inhibits drainage.

For the sinus and chest congestion that accompanies a cold or flu, a eucalyptus steam inhalation works well to loosen the congestion. Hot ginger or peppermint tea also helps to thin mucus, and spicy foods such as jalapeno peppers and horseradish will provide immediate relief. It's also helpful to flush your sinuses a couple of times a day with a simple warm water saline rinse, described in Chapter 7.

Avoid nasal decongestants, which can easily result in dependency on the product. When used for more than a couple of days, nasal decongestants tend to lose their effectiveness. People often increase their usage, and the congestion continues to worsen, resulting in a cycle that can be difficult to break. Oral decongestants almost always contain pseudoephedrine, which can have serious side effects such as agitation, drowsiness, and changes in heart rate and blood pressure. Some natural decongestants contain the Chinese herb ephedra, which has similar side effects when used in excess, and should be used with caution.

Cough suppressant remedies should not be used for coughs that are productive—in other words, a cough that is bringing up mucus. Coughing is the body's way of preventing mucus from accumulating in the lungs. Instead, use herbs such as anise, licorice root, and thyme that help to thin mucus, which makes it easier to cough up. Painful coughing is often a sign that mucus needs to be loosened. Warm steam inhalations can help, as can chest rubs with menthol-containing essential oils such as peppermint and eucalyptus. A dry, hacking cough that isn't productive can also be eased with warm steam inhalations and essential oil chest rubs, and using a cough syrup that includes wild cherry bark can calm the coughing spasms.

Use Antibiotics Only When Necessary

In general, you should never take antibiotics for a simple cold or flu. The only exception is if you come down with a secondary bacterial infection, such as bronchitis or pneumonia. Colds and flus are caused by viruses, not bacteria, and antibiotics are not effective against viruses. The over-prescribing of antibiotics has caused the emergence of strains of deadly super germs that are resistant to many standard antibiotics.

A recent article in the *Journal of the American Medical Association* reported that as many as half of all antibiotic prescriptions written by internal medicine residents were inappropriate. With more than 150 million prescriptions for antibiotics handed out annually, this means that a lot of unneccessary drugs are being taken by the American public. According to the Centers for Disease Control, the more often an antibiotic is used, the more likely bacteria are to develop resistance to it.

Super germs aren't the only danger associated with antibiotics. Every time you take an antibiotic, you're compromising your health by disrupting the delicate balance of friendly bacteria that live in your intestinal tract. Antibiotics are indiscriminate in their killing and wipe out all bacteria, not just disease-causing ones. Common problems that arise from disrupted intestinal flora include digestive disturbances, such as gas and malabsorption, and genitourinary tract infections. More serious health disorders, including elevated levels of harmful cholesterol, PMS and menopausal problems, depressed im - munity, and arthritis, are also associated with antibiotic use.

While few people would dispute the benefits of antibiotics for life-threatening diseases, these powerful drugs should be used appropriately. Appropriate candidates for antibiotic use are those—such as the very young, the very old, and people who are immune-compromised—who are particularly vulnerable to runaway infections. As for the rest of us, antibiotics should be reserved for those times when they are absolutely necessary.

Unfortunately, the reality is that most antibiotics are prescribed for everyday infections, none of which are life threatening, and some of which are not even caused by bacteria. As you now know, the common cold is viral, not bacterial, and is not affected in the least by antibiotics. Yet doctors continue to prescribe antibiotics to treat colds.

If You Do Need Antibiotics

Obviously, there are occasions when antibiotics can be lifesaving. If your doctor prescribes antibiotics for a bacterial infection, be sure to take the full course, even though you may start to feel better before you have finished taking the medication. This ensures that all of the bacteria will be eradicated and won't leave any behind that can mutate into more deadly germs.

If you do need to take antibiotics, there are simple steps you can take to replenish your friendly intestinal flora. It's a good idea to use supplements of beneficial flora during antibiotic treatment and for one month afterward. Take one-half to one teaspoon of a flora supplement that contains both *L. acidophilus* and *Bifidobacterium bifidum* three times a day before meals. Because young children have different concentrations of flora in their intestines, infants should be given one-eighth teaspoon and toddlers one-quarter teaspoon of *Bifidobacterium infantis* three times a day.

Most of the time, you can effectively treat colds and flus with simple home remedies such as the ones you'll find in the next chapter. In contrast to drugs, these natural remedies support your body's attempts at healing and have no dangerous or unpleasant side effects.

CHAPTER 7

HOME REMEDIES FOR COLDS AND FLUS

When I came down with a cold or flu as a child, my mother fed me hot homemade chicken soup to bolster my energy and had me gargle with warm salt water to ease my sore throat. Simple home remedies such as these are often the most effective treatment for relieving the symptoms of a cold or flu. If you do come down with a cold or flu, try these safe, gentle, and effective treatments for easing your discomfort and speeding your recovery.

General Guidelines for Treating Colds and Flus

- **Rest as much as possible.** As soon as you begin to feel cold or flu symptoms, stay home and take it easy. Pushing yourself to remain active will only prolong the virus. In addition to resting, sleep as much as possible to give your immune system the chance to do its job.

- **Drink plenty of fluids.** When you're sick, you need at least two quarts of water daily. Fluids help to thin mucous secretions and aid the body in eliminating toxins. To make plain water more refreshing, add a few slices of fresh lemon or lime.

- **Sip hot herbal teas.** Hot herbal teas loosen congestion and soothe a sore throat. The heat also helps to inhibit viral replication.

- **Eat chicken soup.** As far back as ancient Rome, chicken soup has been recommended for easing respiratory ailments. Recent scientific studies at the University of Nebraska have shown that chicken soup contains anti-inflammatory properties that relieve congestion. Homemade soup is better than canned, and the spicier, the better.

- **Avoid dairy products.** Milk, cheese, and ice cream all increase the production of mucus. Studies have shown that a chemical in milk stimulates the release of histamine, which triggers a runny nose and congestion. The only exception is plain yogurt in small amounts (no more than one cup daily) because it is generally easier to digest and contains beneficial microorganisms.

- **Stay away from refined sweeteners.** Sugar (including sucrose, honey, maple syrup, molasses, fructose, and corn syrup) weakens the immune system and makes it more difficult for your body to overcome a virus. Studies have shown that one serving of a sugary food can reduce the activity of infection-fighting white blood cells by as much as 40 percent. Fruit juices—even unsweetened juices—are high in fructose, which is a simple sugar. Avoid drinking large amounts (more than eight ounces daily) of juice.

- **Eat garlic.** Excellent for fighting the viruses that cause colds and flus, garlic (*Allium sativum*) is a powerful ally for your immune system. Eat one to three cloves of raw garlic daily at the first inkling of a cold or flu. Chop finely and add to hot vegetable or chicken soup just before serving.

- **Take echinacea and elderberry extracts.** These

two herbal cold and flu fighters should be in every home medicine chest. Echinacea (*Echinacea spp.*) stimulates your immune system to overcome the infection, and elderberry (*Sambucus nigra*) prevents the virus from rep-licating. Take one-half teaspoon of echinacea extract and one teaspoon of elderberry extract four times a day in one-quarter cup of warm water for up to ten days.

- **Use zinc lozenges.** Zinc stops viral reproduction in the throat when the throat tissues are saturated with it. Take 15–25 mg of zinc gluco-nate in lozenge form every two hours (up to ten lozenges a day) for up to one week.

- **Increase vitamin C intake.** Take 2,000–5,000 mg of vitamin C daily. High doses of vitamin C have been shown to shorten the duration of the common cold.

- **Use fever to your advantage.** There's no need to lower your temperature unless you have a fever of 102°F or higher. A fever is your body's way of killing the virus. In fact, a slight fever is desirable because it will help you overcome the virus more quickly.

When to Call Your Doctor

While most colds and flus can be safely treated at home, you should contact your healthcare prac-titioner for guidance if you experience the fol-lowing symptoms, because they may indicate a more serious infection:

- Fever over 102°F

- Shortness of breath or a persistent, uncontrol-lable cough

- Persistently coughing up green or yellow mucus

(Upper respiratory infections can sometimes turn into pneumonia; symptoms include a cough accompanied by a fever over 102°F, or a cough with shortness of breath and bloody, brown, or green mucus.)

- A sore throat that lasts for longer than one week

- A fever with a sore throat and swollen glands under the jaw (may indicate strep throat)

Chill-Chasing Herbal Tea

Warming herbs such as ginger (*Zingiber officinalis*) and cinnamon (*Cinnamomum zelandicum*) make delicious teas for helping to chase the chills that often accompany a cold or flu. Ginger, cinnamon, and licorice root (*Glycyrrhiza glabra*) have infection-fighting properties, and lemon adds a healthy dose of vitamin C. Honey has expectorant action and helps to loosen congestion.

2 tablespoons grated
fresh ginger root

1 stick cinnamon bark

2 teaspoons licorice root

½ lemon

1 tablespoon honey (or to taste)

3 cups water

To make a tea, simmer two tablespoons of fresh grated ginger root, one stick of cinnamon, and two teaspoons of dried licorice root in three cups of water in a covered pot over low heat for ten minutes. Remove from heat and allow to steep for an additional ten minutes. Add the juice of one-half lemon, and one tablespoon of honey (or more as desired). Drink the tea hot, one-half cup to one cup up to three times a day.

Lower a Fever with Yarrow-Elderflower-Peppermint Tea

A tea made from yarrow, elderflower, and peppermint promotes sweating and helps to safely lower a fever. Pour three cups of boiling water over two teaspoons each of dried yarrow, elderflower, and peppermint. Cover, and steep for fifteen minutes. Strain, and drink the hot tea in quarter-cup doses every fifteen minutes until the fever subsides. To subdue the bitter flavor, add lemon and honey to taste.

Cool a Fever with a Sponge Bath

To relieve the discomfort of a fever, use a cooling yarrow-lavender sponge bath. Yarrow (*Achillea millefolium*) has anti-inflammatory and antimicrobial properties, and lavender (*Lavendula angustifolia*) is calming, cooling, and soothing. Make a strong yarrow tea by pouring two cups of boiling water over three tablespoons of dried yarrow flowers. Cover, and steep for twenty minutes. Strain, and dilute the tea with an additional two cups of tepid water. Add three drops of lavender essential oil.

Wring out a washcloth in the lukewarm herb water and gently sponge the entire body, or at least the forehead, the back of the neck, the insides of the elbows, the backs of the knees, and the soles of the feet. This can be repeated as often as needed.

Sweat Out a Fever

When your body is confronted with a virus, it mounts a fever to kill the invader, and when the mission has been accomplished, it breaks into a sweat to cool down naturally.

At the first sign of a cold or flu, an old-fashioned sweating cure can aid your body's efforts. By drinking hot herbal tea, taking a hot bath, and covering yourself with blankets until you break into a sweat, you can help raise your body temperature and speed your recovery.

Make a pot of ginger tea by simmering two tablespoons of fresh ginger root in three cups of water in a covered pot for ten minutes. Ginger helps to increase sweating by stimulating circulation and dilating the capillaries at the surface of the skin. Draw a hot bath and soak for fifteen minutes while sipping one or two cups of ginger tea.

Towel dry, put on cotton pajamas, and get into bed and cover up with several blankets. Although you may feel uncomfortable, stay under the blankets until you naturally break into a sweat and the fever begins to subside. Take a tepid bath, dry off, and go to sleep.

Ease Congestion with Eucalyptus Steam

A steam inhalation using tea tree, eucalyptus, and peppermint essential oils helps to loosen chest congestion and ease coughs. Tea tree oil has antiviral and antibacterial properties, eucalyptus oil helps to drain mucous congestion and is antibacterial, and peppermint oil is rich in menthol, which helps to calm spasmodic coughs.

To make a steam inhalation, bring two quarts of water to a boil. Pour into a large heat-proof bowl, and add two drops each of tea tree, eucalyptus, and peppermint essential oils to the steaming hot water. Cover your head and the bowl with a bath towel and breathe in the vapors for ten minutes, being careful to not burn yourself with the steam.

For additional relief from congestion, follow the steam inhalation with a chest and back massage using the same essential oils. Make an aromatherapy massage oil by adding twenty drops of tea tree, twenty drops of eucalyptus, and five drops of peppermint oil to four ounces of almond oil.

Relieve Achiness with an Epsom Salts Bath

To ease the misery of the muscle aches and pains that often accompany the flu, try soaking in an Epsom salts bath. Epsom salts are a rich source of magnesium, which is an excellent muscle relaxant and sedative for the nervous system. Soaking in a hot bath with Epsom salts relaxes muscles, and adding rosemary and lavender essential oils adds additional pain-relieving benefits. As a beneficial side effect, this bath will also help you sleep better. Enough magnesium is absorbed through the skin during an Epsom salts bath to have a relaxing effect on the body and mind.

Add two to three cups of Epsom salts (available at pharmacies) to a bathtub and fill the tub with comfortably hot water. If you want to use essential oils, add five drops each of eucalyptus and lavender oils to the Epsom salts, stir well, and then add to the water. Remain in the tub for at least twenty minutes or longer if desired. Continue to add warm water as needed to keep the bath at a comfortable temperature. Gently towel dry after emerging from the bath and rest.

Soothe a Sore Throat with Ginger Tea

A tasty herbal tea made from marshmallow, ginger root, and peppermint is helpful for easing the pain of a sore throat. Marshmallow (*Althaea officinalis*) contains a water-soluble fiber called mucilage that soothes irritated throat tissues, and ginger (*Zingiber officinalis*) and peppermint (*Mentha piperita*) both help to relieve inflammation.

Make a tea by simmering one tablespoon each of marshmallow root and chopped fresh ginger root in three cups of water in a covered pot for five minutes. Remove from heat, add two teaspoons of peppermint, cover, and steep for an additional ten minutes. Strain, sweeten if desired, and drink as often as desired.

Sage-Lavender-Salt Sore Throat Gargle

A warm gargle made from sage, lavender, and salt temporarily relieves sore throat pain and promotes healing. Sage (*Salvia officinalis*) contains astringent compounds, lavender (*Lavendula angustifolia*) is anti-inflammatory, and salt is mildly antiseptic. Pour one cup of boiling water over one teaspoon each of dried sage leaves and lavender blossoms, cover, and steep for fifteen minutes. Strain, add one-half teaspoon of sea salt, and gargle with the warm solution several times a day.

Nasal Rinse for Easier Breathing

Nasal rinsing is an ancient Ayurvedic cleansing practice that is helpful for treating colds and sinus congestion. Warm, slightly salty water flushes excess mucus from the nose and sinuses, and the salt gently tightens swollen mucous membranes, which temporarily makes it easier to breathe. Small ceramic pots with spouts called neti pots are especially made for nasal rinsing and are available at natural food stores. You can also use a small cup, but a neti pot is easier to work with. It's essential to use comfortably warm water with just the right amount of salt to soothe, not irritate, tender mucous membranes.

Thoroughly dissolve one-quarter teaspoon of sea salt in one cup of warm water. If you are using a neti pot, lean over the sink, insert the spout of the pot into one nostril, and allow the water to flow through the nostril and out of the opposite nostril or your mouth. If you are using a cup, lean over the sink, close one nostril with your finger, sniff the water into your open nostril, and spit the water out of your mouth. Whichever technique you are using, repeat to the opposite side. Repeat up to four times a day.

Herbal Cough Syrup

If a cough is productive (bringing up mucus), it shouldn't be suppressed because your body is getting rid of excess mucus and preventing mucus from accumulating in your lungs. An herbal cough syrup can help your body's efforts. Thyme (*Thymus vulgaris*), licorice root (*Glycyrrhiza glabra*), peppermint (*Mentha piperita*), and anise seed (*Pimpinella anisum*) loosen mucous congestion and relax the respiratory tract. Honey also thins mucus secretions, soothes irritated mucus membranes, and preserves the cough syrup. For a more potent cough syrup to ease spasmodic coughs, add wild cherry bark (*Prunus serotina*), which has powerful sedative action.

To make the cough syrup, gently simmer one tablespoon each of licorice root and crushed anise seeds in two cups of water in a covered pot for fifteen minutes. If you're using wild cherry, add one tablespoon of dried bark and simmer with the licorice root and anise seeds. Remove from heat, add one tablespoon each of dried thyme and peppermint leaves, cover, and steep for one hour. Strain, and add one cup of honey, warming the tea gently if necessary to completely dissolve the honey. Store in a covered glass jar in the refrigerator (it will keep for at least three months). Take one teaspoon as often as needed to relieve a cough.

Soothe Bronchitis with Mullein Tea

Mullein leaves (*Verbascum thapsus*) have been

used for centuries in Ayurvedic, Native American, and European herbalism for the treatment of colds, coughs, sore throats, and bronchitis. The velvety leaves are rich in mucilage, a gelatinous substance that soothes irritated mucous membranes and bronchial passages.

To make a tea, combine mullein with an equal part of marshmallow root, which also contains mucilage and has a slightly sweet taste. This helps to mellow the taste of the mullein leaves, which are slightly bitter and astringent. Pour three cups of boiling water over one tablespoon each of dried mullein leaf and marshmallow root. Cover, and steep for fifteen minutes. Sweeten with honey, if desired, and drink three cups a day until symptoms are relieved.

Loosen Chest Congestion with Mustard

A mustard plaster can loosen deep lung congestion and help to relieve bronchitis. Use caution to avoid leaving the plaster on for too long, because it can blister the skin.

To make a mustard plaster, mix together one tablespoon of powdered mustard, four tablespoons of flour, and enough hot water to make a thin paste. Spread the paste onto a thin cotton tea towel and fold the towel to make a flat pack, with the mustard paste on the inside of the pack. Because mustard stains, be sure to use an old towel.

Place the pack on the chest and cover with a thick towel. Allow the plaster to remain in place for about twenty minutes, but lift a corner of the plaster every few minutes to make sure that the plaster is not burning the skin. A feeling of warmth and a healthy pink color are signs that the plaster is working, but remove the plaster immediately if an uncomfortable burning sensation, redness, or irritation develops.

How to Treat Sinusitis

Sinus infections can be difficult to eradicate because the damp, dark recesses of the sinus cavities provide a perfect breeding ground for infectious microorganisms. An important job of the sinuses is to produce mucus, which cleanses, warms, and moistens the air that we breathe. But when the passages that drain the sinuses swell (such as occurs with a cold or flu) fluids back up into the sinuses and can become infected by microorganisms, usually bacteria.

Symptoms of sinusitis include nasal congestion, pressure or pain in the sinuses, headache, and a yellowish-green mucous discharge. To get rid of a sinus infection, you need to relieve the congestion and eliminate the invading microorganisms. Here's what you should do:

- To ease pain and encourage drainage, apply hot compresses to your sinuses. Add three drops of eucalyptus essential oil to a small basin of hot water. Soak a thick, cotton washcloth in the water and place it over your sinuses, being careful to not burn yourself. Rewet the cloth when it cools and reapply for a total of ten minutes. Repeat several times a day as desired. Eucalyptus (*Eucalyptus globulus*) helps to decongest stuffy nasal passages and the heat eases pain.

- To relieve congestion, use a steam inhalation twice daily. Hot steam loosens and thins mucus so that it can be expelled, and adding anti-microbial essential oils to the steam helps to fight infection. Make a steam inhalation by pouring one and one-half quarts of boiling water into a heat-proof bowl. Add five drops of eucalyptus essential oil and two drops of peppermint essential oil. Make a towel tent over your head and the bowl and breathe in the steam for ten minutes, taking care to not burn yourself with the steam. Eucalyptus has powerful antimicrobial properties, and peppermint (*Mentha piperita*) has a strong penetrating fragrance that helps to open sinus passages.

- Drink plenty of fluids to thin mucous secretions. Hot liquids are especially helpful—try peppermint tea for its decongesting properties, and vegetable or chicken soup with a clove of chopped raw garlic to fight the infection.

- Take echinacea to strengthen your immune response, one-half teaspoon of liquid extract three times a day for ten days. Repeat the dosage after a three-day break if necessary.

How to Treat a Middle-Ear Infection

Middle-ear infections send more parents running to doctors and emergency rooms than any other childhood illness. Antibiotics are almost always prescribed, despite well-documented research that shows that antibiotics are not effective and can make the problem worse.

Middle ear infections cause intense pain and may be accompanied by fever and chills. These infections are caused by viruses or bacteria and usually occur following an upper respiratory illness. Infectious microorganisms can easily travel from the throat to the middle ear, and congestion associated with a cold or flu causes fluid to build up in the middle ear. The warm, dark, moist environment of the middle ear provides a perfect environment for microorganisms to grow.

Try these safe, natural remedies for relieving an ear infection:

- Garlic oil ear drops fight the infection directly in the ear. Some natural foods stores carry garlic oil. To make your own, mince one large bulb of fresh garlic and place in a double boiler with enough olive oil to cover the garlic by one inch. Cover the pot, and warm gently over low heat for one hour. Cool, strain the oil through several layers of cheesecloth, and refrigerate in a covered glass jar for up to one month. To use the oil, warm a small amount in a metal spoon over a candle flame to a comfortable temperature (test the oil on the back of your hand to make sure that it isn't too hot). Place two drops into the ear canal with an ear dropper and plug with a cotton ball. Repeat every hour as needed until symptoms subside.

- You can also use mullein flower oil ear drops, which are available in natural foods stores. Mullein (*Verbascum thapsus*) relieves inflammation and is traditionally used for earaches.

- Place a hot water bottle wrapped in a towel over the ear to help ease pain.

- Give echinacea extract to boost immune function. Children over age six can be given one-half teaspoon three times a day, while children under age six can be given one-quarter teaspoon three times a day.

While ear infections are rarely a medical emergency, they do cause significant pain. Follow the remedies given above to ease the pain, and if the infection does not begin to subside within twenty-four hours, consult your healthcare practitioner.

CHAPTER 8

HOW TO BUY AND USE SUPPLEMENTS AND HERBS

I n reading this book, you've learned a great deal about the dietary supplements and herbs that bolster immunity and help to protect you from colds and flus. But choosing among the vast array of products that are available can be confusing. In this chapter, you'll find the information you need to buy, store, and use supplements and herbs with confidence.

Buying and Storing Supplements

Walk down the aisle of any natural foods store, supermarket, or drugstore, and you're likely to find hundreds of nutritional and herbal supplements. When choosing between various brands of supplements, you'll invariably see a wide variation in price. The more expensive brands are not necessarily better, but just as with most other things in life, there is usually a correlation be - tween price and quality. In other words, you generally get what you pay for. One indication of higher quality products is that they are usually made without artificial colors, preservatives, or sugar.

It's important to buy supplements in a form that appeals to you. Some people have trouble swallowing large vitamin tablets. Hard tablets can also be difficult to digest, and your body may not break them down efficiently. Capsules of powdered supplements or softgel capsules are usually easier to digest.

To maintain the potency of your supplements, you should store them in a cool, dark, dry place, such as a kitchen cabinet away from the stove. Don't keep them in the bathroom, because the high levels of humidity will affect potency. Most supplements should not be refrigerated, with the exception of gel capsules of oil-based supplements, such as vitamin E. The best way to store bulk dried herbs (such as those bought loose for tea) is in a tightly lidded glass jar, away from heat and light.

A Few Words about Herbs

Herbs are available dried for use in teas and also in the form of liquid extracts, capsules, and tablets. Basically, you can use the form that most appeals to you. Teas are inexpensive and are the traditional way of using herbs, but they also entail the most time-consuming method of preparation, they don't extract all of the medicinal properties of certain herbs, and some herbs don't make a pleasant-tasting tea. However, hot herbal teas (such as ginger) are excellent for alleviating the chills of a cold or flu.

When buying loose dried herbs, choose those that have a vibrant color and strong aroma and flavor. Heat, light, and oxygen destroy the medicinal properties of herbs. To maintain the freshness and potency of herbs, store them tightly covered in a glass jar in a cool, dark, dry place (not in the refrigerator) and use them within six months.

Liquid herbal extracts are a combination of water and food-grade alcohol. They contain a broader spectrum of the healing properties of a plant than teas because certain compounds will dissolve in alcohol, but not in water. Alcohol-free extracts are made with vegetable glycerin for people who wish to avoid alcohol, but glycerin is not as effective at dissolving some compounds. Extracts are convenient to take and are highly concentrated—one-half teaspoon of liquid extract is equivalent to approximately one cup of herbal tea. Liquid extracts will retain their potency for at least three years if stored in a cool, dark place.

While capsules and tablets may be convenient to take, these forms are often the least potent because they are so highly processed. Be sure to buy capsules only from a reputable manufacturer and use them within a couple of months. Tablets can be difficult to digest and can pass through the digestive system intact. But some herbs are excellent in tablet form— particularly those made as lozenges, which are designed to be slowly dissolved in the mouth for soothing a sore throat.

Liquid extracts and capsules are both available in standardized extracts, which indicate that the herb is processed to contain a specific amount of what is currently believed to be the herb's primary active ingredient. There are a variety of methods that manufacturers use to standardize an herbal extract, including adding high concentrations of the purified active ingredient and removing what are thought to be unimportant constituents.

Standardized extracts were created to provide consistent results for scientific studies, because plants vary in potency according to how they are grown, harvested, and processed. Some batches of herbs may not contain enough of the active compounds to be effective, and standardization eliminates this problem. However, many herbalists believe that there may be other constituents in an herb that are just as important as the identified active ingredient—including compounds that provide support for the active compound and help to buffer any side effects.

For general use, you can try first using a whole herb extract, and if you don't get the results you want after a month, then switch to a standardized extract and see if there is a noticeable difference. If you are in doubt, consult a qualified herbalist for guidance.

How to Take Supplements

To obtain the maximum benefit from the supplements and herbs that you take, it's helpful to follow a few simple guidelines. Most supplements are assimilated best when taken with, or just after, a meal. This is especially true for supplements that are better absorbed with a meal containing some fat, including vitamins A, D, and E.

Taking supplements with meals also helps to prevent the digestive upset that can occasionally occur if you take supplements on an empty stomach. If you are taking liquid herbal supplements, however, they seem to be best absorbed on an empty stomach. Take them a few minutes before a meal and dilute the dosage with a small amount of water or juice to make them more palatable.

It's also best to divide up supplement dosages so that you are taking them two or three times a day instead of all at once. This provides your body with a consistent supply of nutrients throughout the day, improves absorption, and minimizes the amount that is excreted. To gain the maximum benefit from nutritional supplements, you need to take them consistently. One way to remember to take supplements is to establish a specific time for taking them, for example, immediately after meals. It often takes a month or two to obtain the full benefits of supplements that are taken to strengthen the immune system; for herbs, it can take three months or even longer.

Some supplements, such as herbal products, tend to vary greatly in potency. If you're uncertain about how much you should take, it is safe to follow the manufacturer's recommendations on the label.

CONCLUSION

You now have a good understanding of how cold and flu viruses operate, and how your immune system works to ward off invading micro-organisms and strives to keep you healthy. It probably comes as no surprise that colds and flus are the most common illnesses that afflict us, and you've probably suffered from your share of these widespread ailments. With the information in this book, you now have a variety of powerful, natural ways that you can protect yourself and lower your risks of coming down with a cold or flu, even if it seems that everyone around you is getting sick.

Because of the many forms that viruses take and the ease with which they mutate, it's doubtful that science will ever be able to come up with a vaccine against the common cold, and vaccines against the flu don't offer complete protection. But as you've learned, there are many steps that you can take, beginning today, to protect yourself from viruses and to bolster your immune system. By putting the information in this book into practice, you will not only be defending yourself against colds and flus, but you'll be improving your overall health and well-being, as well.

SELECTED REFERENCES

Bauer R, et al. Influence of echinacea extracts on phagocytotic activity. *Zeitschrift fur Phytotherapie*, 1989; 10: 43–48.

Braunig B., et al. Echinacea purpureae radix for strengthening the immune response in flu-like infections. *Zeitschrift fur Phytotherapie*, 1992; 13: 7–13.

Chang HM, But PH, editors. *Pharmacology and Applications of Chinese Materia Medica.* Yeung S, et al., translators. Singapore: World Scientific; 1987, vol. 2.

De Flora S, Grassi C, and Carati L. Attenuation of influenza-like symptomatology and improvement of cell-mediated immunity with long-term N-acetylcysteine treatment. *European Respiratory Journal*, 1997; 10: 1535–1541.

Gorton HC, Jarvis K. The effectiveness of vitamin C in preventing and relieving the symptoms of virus-induced respiratory infections. *Journal of Manipulative and Physiological Therapeutics*, Oct 1999; 22(8): 530–3.

Graham NM, Burrell CJ, Douglas RM, et al. Adverse effects of aspirin, acetaminophen, and ibuprofen on immune function, viral shedding, and clinical status in rhinovirus-infected volunteers. *Journal of Infectious Diseases*, Dec 1990; 162(6): 1277–82.

Josling P. Preventing the common cold with a garlic supplement: a double-blind, placebo-controlled survey. *Advances in Therapy,* Jul–Aug 2001; 18(4): 189–93.

Mossad SB, Macknin ML, Medendorp SV, et al. Zinc gluconate lozenges for treating the common cold. A randomized, double-blind, placebo-controlled study. *Annals of Internal Medicine,* 1996; 125: 81–88.

Prasad AS, Fitzgerald JT, Bao B, et al. Duration of symptoms and plasma cytokine levels in patients with the common cold treated with zinc acetate. *Annals of Internal Medicine,* 2000; 133: 245–252.

Van Straten M, Josling P. Preventing the common cold with a vitamin C supplement: A double-blind, placebo-controlled survey. *Advances in Therapy,* May–June 2002; 19(3): 151–9.

Yunde H, Guoliang M, Shuhua W, et al. Effect of radix astragali seu hedysari on the interferon system. *Chinese Medical Journal,* 1981; 94 (1): 35–40.

Zakay-Rones Z, Varsano N, Zlotnik M, et al. Inhibition of several strains of influenza virus in vitro and reduction of symptoms by an elderberry extract (*Sambucus nigra* L.) during an outbreak of influenza B Panama. *The Journal of Alternative and Complementary Medicine,* 1995; 1: 361–9.

OTHER BOOKS AND RESOURCES

Challem J. *The Inflammation Syndrome: The Complete Nutritional Program to Prevent and Reverse Heart Disease, Arthritis, Diabetes, Allergies, and Asthma.* Hoboken, N.J.: John Wiley and Sons, 2003.

Murray, N, and Pizzorno, J. *Encyclopedia of Natural Medicine,* revised second edition. Rocklin, CA: Prima Publishing, 1998.

Vukovic, L. *Herbal Healing Secrets for Women.* Paramus, NJ: Prentice Hall, 2000.

Vukovic, L. *14-Day Herbal Cleansing.* Paramus, NJ: Prentice Hall, 1998.

GreatLife Magazine
Consumer magazine with articles on vitamins, minerals, herbs, and foods.
Available for free at many health and natural food stores.

Let's Live Magazine
Consumer magazine with emphasis on the health benefits of vitamins, minerals, and herbs.

Customer service:
1-800-676-4333
P.O. Box 74908
Los Angeles, CA 90004
Subscriptions: 12 issues per year, $19.95 in the U.S.; $31.95 outside the U.S.

Physical Magazine

Magazine oriented to body builders and other serious athletes.

Customer service:
1-800-676-4333
P.O. Box 74908
Los Angeles, CA 90004

Subscriptions: 12 issues per year, $19.95 in the U.S.; $31.95 outside the U.S.

The Nutrition Reporter™ newsletter

Monthly newsletter that summarizes recent medical research on vitamins, minerals, and herbs.

Customer service:
P.O. Box 30246
Tucson, AZ 85751-0246
e-mail: jack@thenutritionreporter.com
www.nutritionreporter.com

Subscriptions: $26 per year (12 issues) in the U.S.; $32 U.S. or $48 CNC for Canada; $38 for other countries.

INDEX

Acetaminophen, 55

Ajoene, 42

Alcohol, 20

Alkylamides, 26

Allicin, 42, 44

Alliin, 42

Allinase, 42

Amino acids, 42

Anise, 56, 68

Antibiotics, 24, 42,
    57–59

Antibodies, 6, 19

Antibody-mediated
    immune response,
    19

Antigens, 16, 18, 19

Antihistamines, 47, 55

Antimicrobial
    chemicals, 11

Antioxidants, 47, 50

Ascorbic acid. *See*
    Vitamin C.

Aspirin, 55

Asthma, 4

Astragalus, 21, 30–35
    compounds in, 32
    dosage, 34

recipes, 34–35

research, 33–34

*Astragalus
    membranaceous.
    See* Astragalus.

B cells. *See*
    B lymphocytes.

B lymphocytes, 16, 19

Bacteria, 57, 58

Basophils, 16

Baths, 66
    See also Sponge
    baths.

*Bifidobacterium
    bifidum,* 58

*Bifidobacterium
    infantis,* 58

Bioflavonoids, 38

Bone marrow, 14

Bronchitis, 4, 57, 68,
    69

Candidiasis, 28

Cell-mediated
    immune response,
    18

Centers for Disease Control, 7, 8
Cherry bark, 56, 68
Chest rubs, 56
Chinese medicine, 21, 30–31
Cichoric acid, 25–26
Cinnamon, 63
Cleanliness, 11
Colds, 3–4, 9–10, 60–68
  prevention, 9–10
  symptoms, 4
  treatment, 60–68
Collagen, 47
Complement fractions, 15, 17
Compresses, 70, 72
Copper, 52
Cough suppressants, 56
Cough syrup, 56, 68
Coughing, 9, 56

Dairy products, 61
Diallyl sufide, 42
Diet, 19–20, 52
Disinfectants, 11–12
Doctors, when to call, 62–63, 72
Doorknobs, 10
Drugs, recreational, 20
Ear infections, 4, 71–72
  treatment, 71–72

Echinacea, 21–30, 61–62, 71, 72
  choosing, 29–30
  compounds in, 25–26
  dosage, 28–29
  history of use, 22–24
  research, 27–28
  side effects, 29
Echinacea spp. See Echinacea.
Echinacoside, 25–26
Eggs, 8
Elder, 36
  flowers, 37, 55, 64
Elderberries, 36–39, 61–62
  dosage, 39
  recipes, 39
  research, 37–38
  side effects, 39
Eosinophils, 16
Ephedra, 56
Epsom salts, 66
Essential oils, 11–12, 65
Eucalyptus, 11–12, 56, 65, 70
Exercise, 20
Eyes, 10

Fatigue, 19
Fats, 20
Fennel, 45

Fever, 18, 62, 64
Flu, 3, 5–10, 60–68
    epidemics, 5–6
    incubation, 7
    mutations, 6–7
    prevention, 9–10
    symptoms, 5
    treatment, 60–68
    types, 6
    vaccine, 7–8
Fruits, 19, 48, 49

Gargling, 67
Garlic, 39–45, 61,
    71–72
    compounds in,
        41–42
    dosage, 45
    fresh, 41–45
    history of, 39–40
    odor, 41, 45
    recipes, 44–45
    research, 42–43
    supplements, 45
Germanium, 42
Ginger, 56, 63, 66–67
Glucose, 47
Glutathione, 50
Glycosides, 42

Hand washing, 10, 11,
    12
Hemagglutinin, 37
Herbs, 60, 63, 74–77
    forms, 74–76

    storage, 74
    usage, 76–77
Histamines, 61
Honey, 63, 68
Horseradish, 56
Huang qi. *See*
    Astragalus.
Humidification, 10

Immune system, 11,
    14–20
Immunity. *See*
    Specific immunity.
Immunoglobulin A
    (IgA), 32, 33
Immunoglobulin E
    (IgE), 32–33
Immunoglobulin G
    (IgG), 32, 33
Immunoglobulin M
    (IgM), 33
Immunoglobulins,
    32–33
Inflammation, 17–18
Influenza. *See* Flu.
Interferon, 15, 17, 18,
    24, 33, 42
Interleukins, 15

Jalapeno peppers,
    56
Juices, 61

Killer T cells. *See*
    T lymphocytes.
King, John, 23

L. acidophilus, 58

Lavender, 11–12, 64, 67

Leukocytes, 24

Licorice root, 56, 63, 68

Lifestyle, 19–20

Limeys, 46

Lloyd, John Uri, 22–23

Lymphatic system, 15
nodes, 14, 15

Macrophages, 15–16, 17, 24, 28, 32

Madaus, Gerhard, 24

Magnesium, 66

Massages, 65–66

Mast cells, 15

Meyer, H. C. F., 22–23

Meyer's Blood Purifier, 22

Monocytes, 16–17

Mucilage, 66, 69

Mucus, 4, 9, 10, 50, 55, 56, 61, 67, 68, 70

Mullein, 68–69, 72

Mumcuoglu, Madeleine, 37–38

Muscle relaxants, 66

Mustard plaster, 69

NAC. *See* N-acetylcysteine (NAC).

N-acetylcysteine (NAC), 50–52
dosage, 52
research, 50–51
side effects, 52

Nasal decongestants, 56

Nasal rinsing, 67–68

Natural killer cells, 16, 17

Neti pots, 67, 68

Neuraminidase, 37, 38

Neutrophils, 16

Nonspecific immunity, 17

Nose, 10

Orange, 11–12

Over-the-counter medications, 3, 55–56

Pandemic, 6

Parsley, 45

Pauling, Linus, 47

Peppermint, 56, 64, 65, 66, 68, 70, 71

Phagocytes, 17, 47

Plasma cells, 19

Pneumonia, 4–5, 57, 63

Polyacetylenes, 26

Polysaccharides, 25, 32

Protein, 19–20

Pseudoephedrine, 56

Qi, 31

Relaxation, 20

Sage, 67
Saline rinse, 56
Salt, 67
Sambucol, 38, 39
Sambucus nigra. See Elderberries.
Saponins, 32
Scurvy, 46
Selenium, 20, 42
Sinusitis, 4, 70–71
    treatment, 70–71
Sleep, 8, 20, 60, 66
Sneezing, 9
Soap, 11–12
Sore throat, 9, 66, 67
Soup, 35, 61, 71
    chicken, 61, 71
    tonic, 35
Specific immunity, 17, 18
Spleen, 14
Sponge baths, 55, 64
Sprays, antibacterial, 12
Steam inhalations, 56, 65–66, 70
Stress, 20
Sugars, 20, 61
Sulfur compounds, 41, 42

Supplements, 73–77
    buying, 73–74
    storage, 74
    usage, 76–77
Sweating cure, 64–65

T cells. *See* T lymphocytes.
T lymphocytes, 15, 16, 18, 24, 33
Tea tree, 11–12, 65
Teas, 34, 37, 55, 56, 60, 63–64, 68–69, 71
    astragalus, 34
    cinnamon, 63
    elderflower, 37, 55, 64
    ginger, 56, 63, 66–67
    herbal, 60, 63
    mullein, 68–69
    peppermint, 56, 64, 71
    yarrow, 55, 64
Telephones, 10
Thyme, 56, 68
Thymus gland, 14, 15, 52
Tobacco, 20

U.S. Food and Drug Administration, 8

Vaccines, 7–8, 79
Vegetables, 19, 48, 49

Viruses, 3, 6, 9, 57
    spread of, 9
Vitamin A, 20, 42
Vitamin B, 42
    complex, 20
Vitamin C, 20, 42,
    46–49, 62
    dosage, 48, 49
    research, 48–49
    side effects, 49
*Vitamin C and the
    common cold,* 47
Vitamin E, 20, 42
Vitamins, multi
    with mineral
    supplement,
    20, 54

Water, 60

Weather, 10
White blood cells, 9,
    14, 15–16, 18, 19
    See also
    B lymphocytes;
    Natural killer cells;
    T lymphocytes.
World Health
    Organization, 8

Yarrow, 55, 64
Yogurt, 61

Zinc, 20, 52–54
    dosage, 53–54
    lozenges, 53–54,
    62
    research, 53
    side effects, 54

Printed in the USA
CPSIA information can be obtained
at www.ICGtesting.com
JSHW051957150824
68134JS00050B/81

9 781681 6285